DATE DUE

RABIES

RABIES

P. Dileep Kumar

Biographies of Disease
Julie K. Silver, M.D. Series Editor

GREENWOOD PRESS
Westport, Connecticut • London

Library of Congress Cataloging-in-Publication Data

Kumar, P. Dileep, 1962–
  Rabies / P. Dileep Kumar.
    p. ; cm.—(Biographies of disease, ISSN 1940–445X)
  Includes bibliographical references and index.
  ISBN 978-0-313-34524-1 (alk. paper)
  1. Rabies. I. Title. II. Series.
  [DNLM: 1. Rabies. WC 550 K96r 2009]
RA644.R3K86   2009
614.5′63—dc22   2008033711

British Library Cataloguing in Publication Data is available.

Library of Congress Catalog Card Number: 2008033711
ISBN: 978-0-313-34524-1
ISSN: 1940-445X

First published in 2009

Greenwood Press, 88 Post Road West, Westport, CT 06881
An imprint of Greenwood Publishing Group, Inc.
www.greenwood.com

Printed in the United States of America

The paper used in this book complies with the
Permanent Paper Standard issued by the National
Information Standards Organization (Z39.48-1984).

10 9 8 7 6 5 4 3 2 1

Contents

Series Foreword

Every disease has a story to tell: about how it started long ago and began to disable or even take the lives of its innocent victims, about the way it hurts us, and about how we are trying to stop it. In this Biographies of Disease series, the authors tell the stories of the diseases that we have come to know and dread.

The stories of these diseases have all of the components that make for great literature. There is incredible drama played out in real-life scenes from the past, present, and future. You'll read about how men and women of science stumbled trying to save the lives of those they aimed to protect. Turn the pages and you'll also learn about the amazing success of those who fought for health and won, often saving thousands of lives in the process.

If you don't want to be a health professional or research scientist now, when you finish this book you may think differently. The men and women in this book are heroes who often risked their own lives to save or improve ours. This is the biography of a disease, but it is also the story of real people who made incredible sacrifices to stop it in its tracks.

Julie K. Silver, M.D.
Assistant Professor, Harvard Medical School
Department of Physical Medicine and Rehabilitation

Preface

Rabies is a dreaded disease in many parts of the world, causing several thousand deaths each year. Although this infection is rare in the United States, this has only been the case for a few decades. The disease has been carefully controlled through research and vaccination programs. As the pattern of rabies changes in the United States, bats have replaced dogs as the main carriers of the disease. This book aims to examine these changing trends of rabies in the United States and the world.

Rabies is a story of courageous people all over the world. Stories of patients are illustrated in this book, giving a backdrop to the discussion of the various phases of rabies. The chapters are laid out to give the reader a broad scope of the subject. The pathophysiology of the disease is explained through a series of case studies that might interest any one who has a fascination with infectious diseases. Students of biology and microbiology, and anyone interested in science, will find the stories poignant and thought provoking. Those with an interest in medicine will find this book an interesting read. People who travel or have public health concerns in other counties around the world will find this book particularly relevant.

Finally, the book aims to inspire curiosity in readers. A complete list of references is given with sufficient leads for further scholarship. A glossary of important terms used in the book is also given to facilitate understanding.

Introduction

Everyone knows the word "rabid." It is associated with a terrible disease called rabies. Rabid dogs spreading the disease of rabies are a powerful visual statement that evokes terror in humans. Fortunately, the incidence of rabies in the developed world has recently declined, although developing countries still record significant deaths associated with rabies each year.

Ancient historians and physicians recorded the various features of this disease, predominantly the inability of the victim to swallow water, which is known as "hydrophobia." Louis Pasteur, after a series of painstaking experiments in 1885, developed a vaccine to prevent rabies. A cure for rabies is still evasive, but it can be prevented effectively by a series of vaccinations given after exposure. Several international agencies work to control rabies in developing countries where many people die from the disease each year.

This book also details the current state of knowledge in rabies research and various exciting new developments. In 2004, a 15-year-old girl from Wisconsin became the first person in history to survive after contracting full-fledged rabies and not receiving any preventative vaccines. Her survival is attributed to what is known as the "Milwaukee Protocol," which was thoughtfully developed by a group of physicians and researchers.

There have been several cases of tragic deaths due to rabies in travelers, mainly in Europe. Most of the cases arose from lack of awareness of the disease and inadequate prophylaxis after exposure to animals such as stray dogs. Proper education and awareness will help to prevent such eventualities.

Again, rabies, like any disease that scourges society, is comprised of human stories. It is the story about how people fight against the disease and conquer it, how the concerted action of different agencies across the globe in an inter-connected world offers fresh hope to victims, and how new understanding of the disease changes age-old paradigms and beliefs. This is that story of hope and success.

Timeline

3000 B.C.	Dog as an emissary of death in Vedic period of India, possibly oblique reference to rabies.
2300 B.C.	First reference of rabies in Mosaic Esmuna code of Babylon.
1st century	Roman scholar Celsus thinks rabies is caused by saliva of the animal.
Middle Ages	In Europe, peasants prayed to patron saint of rabies, St. Hubert from Liege.
1709	Bat rabies described in Mexico.
1753	Rabies in Virginia in dogs imported from England.
18th-20th century	Belief in the powers of "madstone" that is able to suck the rabies "poison."
18th century	Efficient stray dog control inhibits rabies in several European countries.
1819	Governor General of Canada dies of rabies.

1849	Edgar Allan Poe's mysterious death in Baltimore, rabies considered a possibility recently.
1885	Louis Pasteur's rabies vaccine is efficient in preventing rabies in Joseph Meister after a dog bite.
1885	Newark dog scare. Four American children bitten by a rabid dog sent to Paris to be vaccinated by Pasteur himself.
1903	Negri describes characteristic inclusion bodies in rabies-infected brain.
Early 1900s	Newer inactivation of neural vaccines by Fermi and Semple.
1911	First scientific report of bovine rabies from South America transmitted by "vampire bats."
1935	Rabies immunoglobulin proved to be efficient in preventing the disease.
1945	Fox rabies noticed in Texas.
1950s	Introduction of the suckling mouse rabies vaccine.
1953	First reported case of rabies transmitted by bats.
1956	A bat researcher dies in Texas due to rabies presumably contracted from bats from a cave with millions of bats.
1959	Introduction of fluorescent antibody testing for rabies.
1963	Matsumoto observes rabies viral particles using electron microscopy.
1970s	Raccoon rabies spreads along the East coast of the US.
1975	Introduction of human diploid cell vaccine for rabies post exposure prophylaxis.
1978	First field trails of oral rabies vaccine in animals. Prevention of the spread of fox rabies in Switzerland.
1983	Vaccinia-based rabies vaccine for oral immunization of animals developed.
1983	The death of a Peace Corps volunteer in Kenya even after rabies vaccination raises questions about the efficacy of intradermal route and other issues.

1980s and 90s	Sustained campaigns of control of rabies in wild animals prevent spread of the disease in several European countries.
1992	Raccoon rabies spread along the East Coast of US reaches Massachusetts.
1994	Oral rabies vaccine program instituted by the Texas Department of Health in wild animals to prevent the spread of rabies.
1994	Prophylactic efforts to prevent rabies after several people were exposed to a rabid kitten in New Hampshire costs $1.5 million.
2004	Multiple organ transplant recipients in four southern states afflicted with rabies from a donor in whom the rabies diagnosis was not made till death.
2004	Wisconsin teenager survives after battling rabies for several weeks in the intensive care unit. Milwaukee protocol where doctors employed 'induced coma' credited with her recovery.
2006	Attempts to cure rabies failed in Indiana and California. They did survive longer than average patients with rabies.
2007	First World Rabies Day launched on September 8, 2007, with the motto "Working together to make rabies history."

1

Rabies and History

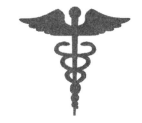

RABIES: AN ANCIENT DISEASE

Rabies is a disease that has frightened civilizations over the centuries. It has been recognized since ancient times. The bite of a rabid animal guaranteed certain death. The end was painful, with the victim being unable to swallow water for days. Even the sight of water produced painful contractions of the laryngeal muscles, reflexively causing severe agony. This characteristic symptom is called hydrophobia (fear of water) and has become synonymous with the disease. The victim then slowly slipped into a coma because of the combination of dehydration and exhaustion.

Several ancient civilizations have references to this devastating disease. The origin of the word rabies could either be from the Sanskrit word, *rabhas*, which means "to do violence," or from the Latin *rabere*, meaning "to rage or rave." The Vedic period in India (3000 B.C.) has the god of death attended by a dog as the emissary of death. The first reference to rabies, describing its lethality in dogs and human beings, can be found in the Mosaic Esmuna code of Babylon written during 2300 B.C. Babylonians made the owner of a rabid dog pay a fine if his dog bit and transmitted rabies to another person. Greeks were also aware of the disease and coined the term *lyssa* for rabies, derived from the word *lud*, which means "violent" in Greek. The Roman scholar

Celsus was the first to describe human rabies in the first century A.D. He thought the saliva of the biting animal caused the infection. There were references to rabies in Ancient Egypt as well. The Egyptian god Sirius was depicted in the form of a mad dog. The constellation Canis Major that includes Sirius appears in the sky during late summer when rabies is more likely to be prevalent.

The disease and its barbaric cures have evoked terror in public minds throughout the centuries. The Roman scholar Celsus assumed that people could get infected with rabies. He also suggested several cures for rabies. One was to hold the affected person underwater to cure the "hydrophobia." If the victim was not drowned by this maneuver, the individual died of hydrophobia. Cauterization of the bite wounds with a red-hot poker was a favorite treatment throughout the Middle Ages. Most of the time these aggressive cauterizations resulted in widespread damage of the tissue and infections.

"Hair of the dog" was a ritual that was practiced with several variations all over the world. This practice consisted of applying the hair of the rabid dog to the victim's wound in the belief that it would cure rabies. Alternatively, eating the hair, heart, or liver of the animal was also practiced based on the "like cures like" principle. In modern times, the phrase "hair of the dog" refers to the practice of curing an alcoholic hangover by ingesting more alcohol in the morning. This term originated from the rabies treatment of the Middle Ages. In medieval Europe, farmers prayed to St. Hubert, patron saint of rabies, to have them spared from the horrible disease. They traveled to Liege, a city in present day Belgium, to pray to the saint. Peasants used iron bars or crosses called "keys" of St. Hubert to protect them from rabies. Patients killed themselves and some individuals were killed by others if bitten by a rabid dog. Some countries even passed laws banning the deliberate killing of people afflicted with rabies.

It is debatable how and when rabies was introduced to the Americas. It is possible that the native bats of the continent carried the virus, as reported by a Spanish bishop of the new world, Petrus Martyr Anglerius. He observed Spanish soldiers suffering from the illness after coming into contact with the bats. Fray Jose Gil Ramirez also described rabies in Mexico in 1709. As for North America, the first reported cases occurred in dogs brought to Virginia from England in 1753.

Madstones (18th to 20th century)

Madstones are a fascinating part of the history of rabies treatment during the colonization of the American West. These stones were used to cure the "madness" of rabies. From the 1800s to the turn of the 20th century, madstones were touted as a popular cure for human rabies. Madstone is a calcified mass derived from the digestive tracts of cud-chewing animals such as deer, goats, and cows. Cud is the food ingested by a ruminant that is regurgitated to be chewed again. Madstone consisted of the animal's fur, plant stalks, and other indigestible matter that the animal had eaten. In many ways it is like a very hard hairball. They are concretions of calcium, deposited layer upon layer around a foreign body in the animal's digestive tract, forming a "stone." This process is similar to an oyster forming a pearl. Nowadays, few hunters examine the stomach contents of deer they kill, but old-timers did in the hopes of finding one of these magical restoratives. Folklorists claim that madstones were more highly prized than rubies because of their supposed curative powers. The best stone was believed to come from the stomach of a white deer.

During the frontier days, people in possession of madstones were well known, and victims of animal bites were often carried long distances for treatment. It is believed that in 1849, after Abraham Lincoln's son Robert was bitten by a rabid dog, the future president took the boy from Springfield, Illinois, to Terre Haute, Indiana, so that a madstone practitioner could treat him. The madstones were owned by certain families, passed on through the generations as family heirlooms, and were believed to possess special powers. Usually the service was free, but owners never loaned out a stone. The user required no special knowledge or power to effect a treatment. The madstone was a treasured possession hidden for safekeeping. Even today, madstones are prized as collector's items.

The rabies treatment began by boiling the madstone in sweet milk or water. The hot stone was then applied directly to the wound caused by the rabid dog. If the dog was actually mad, the stone stuck to the wound and would draw the poison out. The stone was said to become attached to the oozing wound for a variable time without the help of any bandage or tape. There were documentations detailing such attachments lasting for hours or days. The stone was believed to suck out the rabies poison during this period and cure the person of rabies. Supposedly, the porosity of the stone together with the moisture in the wound caused it to adhere to the flesh and presumably draw out the poison (Georgia Department of Human Resources, 2004). Once the body was cleared of the rabies "poison," the stone fell off automatically. The same stone could be reused after boiling it in sweet milk and reapplying to the wound. The milk would turn green from the poison. This process was repeated until the stone no long adhered to the wound, indicating that all the poison had been removed. Madstones were held as "family jewels" and passed down from generation to generation. On February 1, 1805, Essex County, Virginia, reported the sale of a local madstone for a price of $2,000!

Jake Grimes, owner of a madstone in Hutchinson, Kansas, kept a record of everyone who was treated with his stone for a mad animal bite. The individual's age, date, address, and the duration of the treatment in hours was recorded. Most of the people seeking treatment came from within 100 miles or so from Hutchinson. Rarely, patients visited from as far as Texas. A man named S. C. Turnbo described a madstone he found in a deer that was shot on the Eleven Point River in Oregon County, Missouri (Gilmore, 1995). The stone was about 2.5 inches in length, an inch thick, and had "small pimples or cells all over it." Madstones have always been greatly prized by anyone possessing one. Turnbo says that he was offered $200 for his stone, but he refused and gave it to a relative who took it into Indian Territory with him.

Madstones were also used to draw the poison from a snakebite or treat various aches and pains. It is very difficult to ascertain how this stone became part of the treatment of rabies. Early settlers' healthcare relied heavily on folk remedies. Rabies was an incurable disease during that era. People dreaded the disease and wanted to do something to obtain a cure. Reported cures of rabies might have occurred in patients who never had rabies but a syndrome that mimics rabies. This is called pseudo (false) rabies or hysterical rabies. After a bite from a dog (probably not a rabid one) some of the victims develop intense fear of contracting rabies. The person starts showing symptoms of anxiety, difficulty in swallowing, or even spasms. This condition is not lethal and abates by itself, after prompt reassurance or placebo treatment, as might have been provided by a madstone. There is no scientific evidence that such a stone, however porous, could suck out "rabies poison." In any case, the use of madstones appears to have been discredited in the western United States by the end of the 19th century.

Interestingly a similar practice also exists in the Philippines. A black porous stone is applied to the wound in the hope of sucking the rabies poison out of the wound. In a variation of this practice, rural quack doctors also use a corn-shaped horn of the carabao, a domesticated water buffalo common to the Philippines. These practices, known as "tandok," are discredited in modern times, although they are still prevalent among the poor rural populace.

Edgar Allan Poe Mystery

In modern times, rabies has been linked to the cause of death of Edgar Allan Poe (January 19, 1809, to October 7, 1849), who was an American poet, short story writer, editor, and literary critic. He is famous for the American Romantic movement and wrote tales of macabre and mystery. Poe died at the Washington College Hospital in Baltimore on October 7, 1849.

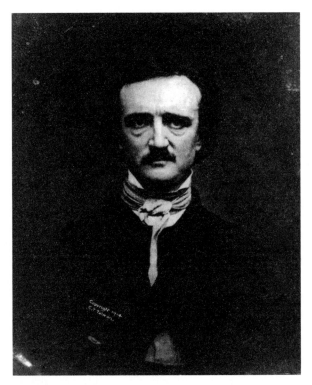

Edgar Allan Poe. (Library of Congress)

Circumstances leading to his death are as mysterious as one of his stories. The prominent theory behind the cause of his death is alcoholism and delirium tremens that can result from withdrawal of alcohol. But in 1995, Dr. Michael Benitez, a cardiologist from the University of Maryland Medical Center at Baltimore, Maryland, came up with a new theory about Poe's demise (Mackowiak, 2007, 250).

Edgar Allan Poe was born to an English actress and an Irish actor. His mother died, presumably of tuberculosis, when he was 2 years old. His father was an alcoholic and Poe himself had a lifelong battle with alcohol problems. He met with several literary successes after the publication of several stories and poems. Poe's first wife, Virginia, apparently died of tuberculosis and the author had to fight bouts of depression as a consequence. In the spring of 1849, he left New York to travel to Richmond where he proposed to his childhood sweetheart. On September 27, 1849, he left Richmond for New York. He never reached New York. Instead, he was found lying unconscious on a wooden plank outside Ryan's Saloon on Lombard Street in Baltimore on

October 3, 1849. How he ended up in Baltimore is still a mystery. His suit was disheveled and he was taken to the Washington College Hospital (now Church hospital).

Dr. Joseph Moran was his personal physician. Poe was delirious and tremulous at the hospital. He had hallucinations and gradually he slipped into a coma. When offered alcohol, he refused it. He also had some relatively lucid periods but later became agitated, combative, and again slipped into a coma. He died on October 7, 1849. Dr Moran's later accounts describe that when offered water he had difficulty in swallowing, which might reflect the hydrophobia seen in rabies. He apparently also had autonomic disturbances such as changes in pulse and pupil size during the hospital stay.

An autopsy was not performed and all of the original charts were lost. Dr. Benitez argues that Edgar Allan Poe died of rabies. The course of his illness fits well with the description of the disease. Rabies was not uncommon during that time in that part of the country. There was no history of exposure such as the bite of a rabid dog. However, between 1977 and 1994, 34 patients developed rabies in the United States but only 9 (27 percent) had evidence of appropriate animal exposure.

The features of Poe's illness do resemble rabies, in which the victim is anxious and delirious initially, progressively becomes agitated and confused, and gradually slips into a coma. The disease is almost universally fatal. The difficulty in swallowing known as hydrophobia is a classical sign of rabies. Even the sight of water can cause severe painful contractions of the muscles of the throat that are responsible for swallowing.

Ontario 1819: Governor General of Canada Dies of Rabies

Charles Lennox, 4th Duke of Richmond and Lennox, was a British soldier and politician and Governor General of British North America. He was born in Scotland and showed a keen interest in the game of cricket. Richmond was active in the Naval Wars with the French and participated in the Napoleonic Wars. In 1815 he was in command of a reserve force protecting the Belgian city of Brussels in case Napoleon won the Battle of Waterloo. In 1818 he was appointed Governor General of upper Canada. The Duke arrived in Quebec in July 1818 to govern British North America.

Richmond took an extensive tour of upper and lower Canada in the summer of 1819. At William Henry (now known as Sorel, southwestern Quebec), which is situated at the confluence of the Richelieu River and the St. Lawrence River, he was bitten by a pet fox (Jackson, 1994). The injury apparently healed and he continued his journey to York (present day Toronto) and Niagara examining the military establishments. He returned to Kingston and planned a leisurely visit to the settlements on the Rideau River. The symptoms of rabies developed during this journey. The only way he could receive medical attention was to sail up the St. Lawrence River. The sight of the vast expanse of water terrified the Governor General. Successive violent fits took hold of him. He was unable to drink or swallow any water. He fought his impulses and tried to make the journey up the river. Eventually, he could take it no longer and begged to be rowed to dry land. He got out of the vessel and ran as far away from the water as possible. On August 28, 1819, he died of extreme agony in a barn a few miles away from a settlement that now bears his name (Richmond, Ontario).

Newark Dog Scare of 1885

While Louis Pasteur perfected his technique of vaccination against rabies in 1885, U.S. scientists watched with intense interest. Pasteur was a prolific scientist dabbling in several research projects. He invented ways to save the silkworm industry and wine production in France. Pasteur's ideas became popular across the Atlantic. The wine farmers in California followed Pasteur's techniques of fermentation. Pasteur obtained several American patents for his technology.

Six children were bitten in Newark, New Jersey, in December 1885 by a stray dog. The dog was rabid and ran through the streets, biting everything in sight: humans, animals, and even inanimate objects. The dog was a large black animal and was thought to have come from the countryside. Seventeen dogs were bitten and 12 of them were killed, whereas the rest were isolated for observation. The dog was finally killed while gnawing and clawing at the door of a house. The dog was so ferocious that even the moldings at the bottom of the door were torn off.

Dr. William O'Gorman, who was keenly watching Pasteur's experiments, thought that sending the children to Pasteur was the only way to save them. He suggested a subscription program if the parents were not able to afford the trip (New York Times, 1885). Within a few hours, the doctor received a collection from the employees of a local manufacturing plant. Within 24 hours, sufficient funds arrived as nickels, dimes, and dollars from ordinary folks. Around $1,000 was raised. A local clothing store offered full winter clothing for the children for the winter voyage. Four children were sent to Paris in a ship with some attendants and a doctor. Parents of two of the bitten children refused to send them. A donation from Andrew Carnegie was also made for the trip to be undertaken. The press loved the story and all of the newspapers of New York competed for the special angles of the account. American newspapers filed breathless day-to-day reports of the fate of the children. Their articles were reprinted in out-of-town papers all across the United States. The trip to Paris by four working class boys was an enormous media sensation. On some days a full 10 percent of the *New York Herald* was used to cover rabies and its stories. All of the four children were given the rabies vaccine by none other than Pasteur himself. Returning from Paris, they remained well, and none contracted rabies. The fate of the two children who did not receive the vaccine is unknown. Upon return to United States, the four treated children were even exhibited for a fee in fares and carnivals as miraculous rabies survivors! Crowds paid 10 cents just to hear the boys tell of their Atlantic voyages and how Pasteur had saved their lives. The episode was not free from controversy; some skeptics argued that there was no rabies in Newark and people were getting a free ride to Paris to meet Pasteur.

RABIES IN POPULAR CULTURE

Old Yeller

In more recent times rabies has been portrayed extensively in pop culture. *Old Yeller* is a touching movie with a dog as the important central character.

Old Yeller is a 1957 film directed by Robert Stevenson and produced by Walt Disney Productions. This movie is based on a book by the same name written by Fred Gipson in 1956. The story is set in post Civil War Texas and centers around a boy and the stray dog he befriends.

The Coates family was poor and lived in rural Texas in the late 1860s. Jim and Katie raised their two sons, Travis and Arliss, in a life filled with struggles and dangers. Fourteen-year-old Travis is left to defend his mother and younger brother when his father leaves for a cattle run. Shortly after, a yellow mongrel dog wanders onto their property uninvited. Arliss, the younger of the boys, immediately takes a liking to him, but Travis does not. Travis, in fact, wants to get rid of the dog. But the dog follows him everywhere—while milking the cows, raising the hogs, and hunting deer. Eventually he realizes the usefulness of having a dog following him during his chores. In one incident, the dog saves little Arliss from a frantic mother bear and her cub. The dog also saves Travis from some wild pigs. Yeller eventually gains Travis' respect and love and the two becomes friends.

The author describes the adventures of Travis and Old Yeller and their resultant friendship in colorful language with a memorable style. The owner of the dog, Mr. Sanderson, was looking for Old Yeller and discovers him at the Coates family farm. Realizing how much the family needs the dog, Mr. Sanderson settles for a toad and a home-cooked meal.

Old Yeller bravely defends and saves Travis and his family from several dangers of the times. He is faithful to the core. He thwarts a group of crazed hogs and diverts the attention of a mad bull and cow. He also saves the mother, Katie, and a neighbor girl, Lisbeth, from the jaws of a rabid gray wolf. But Old Yeller was bitten in this fight and soon contracts rabies. He becomes very sick. Travis is faced with the proposition of ending the life of his very best friend, who has saved the lives of his family many times.

To protect his family, Travis tearfully shoots Old Yeller. His father returns, but Travis is not excited by the new horse that his father brings with him. After listening to the story of Old Yeller, his father reassures Travis that he did the right thing. He also reminds him that a man is often left to make tough decisions that are painful at times. Travis realizes that he has taken the first steps of his journey into manhood. He allows his heart to open up to the horse from his father, and to a young pup that was also a gift.

Old Yeller is a tale chronicling the rites of passage, a coming of age tale in post Civil War Texas. The novelist uses the frightening image of an animal affected by rabies to communicate effectively the dilemmas faced by a teenager growing into an adult. The symptoms of rabies are painted realistically. The painful fact that there is no cure for this dreaded disease stares at the characters and the reader. The helplessness is heartbreaking. This tale has captivated generations of readers.

Rage

Rage is a 1966 movie directed by the Mexican director Gilberto Gazcon. It is a suspenseful drama starring Glenn Ford as Reuben, a doctor who has accepted a job at a construction site in the Deep South after the death of his wife during childbirth. He is angry, alone, and tries to kill his sorrow by turning to alcohol. One day a man appears, stumbling out of the desert and dying from rabies. The rabid dog that bit him follows and manages to bite the doctor. After delivering a baby, Reuben takes off on a mad rush across the desert to find medical aid before rabies can kill him. The grateful Pancho and a prostitute named Perla accompany him. The story depicts his fight to live as time is running out. The absorbing rush to obtain the medication is made more urgent by the rapid fury of the disease.

Cujo

Cujo is a horror novel by Stephen King, originally published by Viking in 1981. The novel was made into a 1983 film of the same name. The middle-class

Trenton family, plagued by financial and marital trouble, and the rural Camber clan are at the center stage of this story. While chasing a rabbit in the fields, Cujo, a St. Bernard dog, is bitten by a bat infected with rabies. Vic Trenton leaves the house on a business trip to Boston and New York, leaving his wife, Donna, and their 4-year-old son, Tad, at home.

Cujo is now rabid, and the dog attacks and kills the Camber's neighbor, Gary Pervier, a WWII hero who is now an alcoholic. Joe, another neighbor, goes to Gary's house and finds him dead. Cujo then kills Joe before he can call for help. Without knowing any of these happenings, Donna and Tad take the family car for repairs to the Camber's barn. The car breaks down when they reach the farm. The rabid Cujo terrorizes the mother and the child, who are then trapped in the car in a 3-day siege. Hunger and thirst cause hallucinations and fantasies of escape during the hottest summer in the village's history. Donna is bitten in the stomach and leg during an escape attempt. The sheriff then arrives at the scene, but is killed by the rabid dog. Vic returns home because Donna was not answering her phone. He reaches the farm. Tad dies of heat stroke inside the car, and Donna finally escapes from the car and kills the rabid dog with a baseball bat.

Cujo is a classical man versus nature story. Nature at its very worst and human beings trying to survive by dogged fighting. The story portrays the transformation of a gentle Cujo into a mad rabid dog on a killing spree. However, the story is not a factual account of the manifestation of a rabid dog. It exaggerates the behavior of a rabid animal. But, it is interesting that a bat gives rabies to the dog in the story, echoing the changing epidemiology of rabies in the United States.

Rabies has also been portrayed in several television features and serials. Many popular medical television serials such as *ER*, *House*, and *Grey's Anatomy* have featured segments mentioning rabies. This fearful disease is a powerful symbol of human kind's frailty, which is very appealing to an audience.

THE RABIES VIRUS

Structure and Classification of Rabies Virus

Rabies is a viral disease spread by animals infected with the rabies virus. The disease is almost always fatal in human beings, and only a few cases of survivors have been recorded. Rabies is an RNA (ribonucleic acid) virus. Viruses are smaller than bacteria, ranging from size 10–300 nm (1 nanometer is a thousand-millionth of a meter). Viruses cannot live independently; they need a living cell for their replication. They are very ingenious, using the host cell's multiplication machinery for their benefit. They use the genetic mechanisms of the living cells of animals and humans to duplicate themselves. Rabies virus belongs to the genus *Lyssavirus* (*lyssa* means rage in Greek), which has seven virus genotypes. *Lyssavirus* belongs to the larger family of *Rhabdoviridae*, which includes other rod-shaped viruses. Of the seven *Lyssavirus* genotypes, rabies is the most important type from an epidemiological point of view. The other six are closely related to rabies and are also capable of causing encephalomyelitis (inflammation of the brain and spinal cord) like the rabies virus. The major genotypes of *Lyssavirus* include rabies virus (genotype 1), Lagos bat virus (genotype 2), Mokola virus (genotype 3), Duvenhage virus (genotype 4), European Bat Lyssaviruses 1 and 2 (genotypes 5 and 6), and Australian Lyssavirus (genotype 7).

Rabies virus is shaped like a bullet, with a round end on one side and a flat end on the other side. The virus has an envelope derived from the host cell. Rabies virus is relatively a simple virus and has only five proteins—N, P, M, G and L (Jackson and Wunner, 2002, 25). N (nucleoprotein) protein is the innermost and protects the RNA structure from any enzymatic damage. P (phosphorylation) protein combines with L protein to form important complexes during the replication of the virus. M (matrix) protein lines the inner membrane of the virus. It also acts as a bridge between the cell membrane and the inside core of the virus. G (surface) protein forms spikes on the outer membrane of the virus. The G protein is important in the attachment (binding) of the virus to a host cell. It also interacts with the rabies antibodies in the host's blood. The L (large) protein also takes part in the replication process of the virus.

Rabies has been known to civilization for thousands of years. In one year, more than 55,000 deaths are believed to be caused by rabies worldwide. In the United States, the incidence has fortunately decreased since the early 1900s. There used to be about 100 cases of rabies each year, mostly acquired from domestic animals. Currently only two or three people die per year because of rabies, usually because the victims fail to seek timely medical care or are unaware of their exposure to the disease.

Sylvatic and Urban Cycles of Rabies

Rabies virus is found in mammals on all continents except Antarctica. Two different cycles of viral transmission occur in nature—urban and sylvatic. Knowledge of the spread of this dreaded disease will provide insight into possible methods of control. Urban rabies is transmitted by domestic animals and sylvatic rabies is spread by various wild animals such as raccoons, skunks, foxes, mongooses, wolves, and bats. The urban infection is a result of the virus

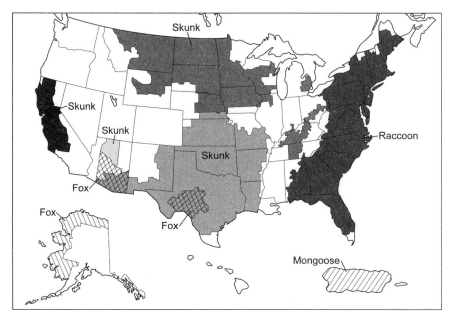

Distribution of major rabies virus variants among wild terrestrial reservoirs in the United States and Puerto Rico. (CDC, 2006. Redrawn by Jeff Dixon)

spreading from the wild cycle. The main reservoir for the urban cycle is the domestic dog. Dog rabies has been eliminated in the United States since the 1960s by the widespread use of canine immunizations. A 10-day observation of the dog is the standard practice in the case of dog bites. If the dog is alive and healthy, rabies is ruled out. Dog rabies is widely prevalent in most of Africa and Asia.

Rabies is maintained in several wild animals. In North America, the major carriers of this virus in the wild are raccoons, skunks, red and gray foxes, coyotes, and insectivorous bat species. The most recent epidemic in the wild was in 1977, when an outbreak of raccoon rabies was detected in an area on the West Virginia/Virginia border. Since then the virus has spread to Ohio in the west; New York, Pennsylvania, Vermont, New Hampshire, and Maine in the north; and Florida in the south. It was estimated that the infection in wild raccoons was spreading at the rate of approximately 18–24 miles each year. Interestingly, the Appalachian Mountains slowed the westward progression of the virus for more than a decade, but it is feared that once the disease reaches the Ohio Valley, there is little to prevent its spread across the nation to the Pacific coast.

Bat rabies is also widespread all over the world and the United States. Since 1980, 30 cases of bat rabies have occurred in the United States. This was 90 percent of all of the rabies cases in the country. Two specific types of bats are implicated in most of the cases: the *Silver Haired* and the *Eastern Pipis-trelle* bats. One reason these bats cause most of the infection is that they have very small teeth; therefore victims can easily overlook the bites.

Exposure to Bats, Virginia 2006

In 2006, the mother of a girl who had attended the Girl Scouts camp at Potomac Woods in Northern Virginia contacted the Girl Scout Council of the nation's capital. The girl had told her mother that the open-air cabin she slept in had bats living in the eaves. Five bats subsequently caught at the camp's shelters tested negative for rabies. Later it was discovered that a few girls apparently touched a bat captured by a counselor, and some girls had not used protective netting around their beds while they slept at night. Girl Scout officials recommended that nearly 1,000 Girl Scouts who may have been exposed to rabies at the camp consider getting rabies vaccinations (the rabies vaccine is effective even after being bitten by a rabid animal). The health department subsequently sent letters to the parents of around 950 girls who attended the camp. The Girl Scouts offered to pay for the vaccine at a rate of approximately $2,000 per person and at a total estimated cost of $2 million. Most parents declined the offer. About 20 campers considered at risk were given the postexposure treatment for rabies with rabies vaccine (Fox News, 2006). Later, camp officials installed screens on windows, doors, and eaves in all 54 of the camp's shelters. The campers were at risk only if they did not use the specially provided nets and either handled a bat or saw a bat nearby after awakening from sleep.

The local health department contacted the parents of each camper who attended Camp Potomac Woods to determine whether any camper may have had contact with a bat and the potential for exposure to rabies. Each parent was mailed a letter explaining the situation, with a questionnaire to ascertain potential exposure. This letter emphasized that "it is unlikely that any camper came in contact with a bat or was exposed to rabies at Camp Potomac Woods" (Virgina Department of Health, 2006). Although the risk of exposure to a bat carrying rabies was small, the health department decided to notify the parents of each camper so that all parents would receive consistent information. The major questions mailed to the parents were as follows:

In regard to her stay at Camp Potomac Woods, does your child remember
(a) Having been bitten by a bat? Yes/No;
(b) Having touched a bat? Yes/No;
(c) Having woken up and found a bat in the cabin where she was sleeping? Yes/No

If the answer to any of these questions was yes, the parent was advised to contact the health department for more information. Some local parents expressed frustration about the difficult decision they faced. The risk, although small, was real and was probably a smart decision on the part of the girls who decided to receive the vaccine because of close contact with the bats.

The Virginia campers are not alone in such rabies scares. At a church camp in Ohio, 440 children and adults from 13 states were investigated for potential exposure to rabies through bats. They slept in a converted movie theater that was found to be full of bats. One woman felt something crawling on her chest, lifted the sheet, and a bat scampered out like a mouse. The woman captured the animal between two flip-flops and threw it outside. She was given postexposure prophylaxis with the rabies vaccine.

This woman's experience posed an obvious risk of an unnoticed scratch or bite from the bat's small, razor-sharp teeth. Because of this, the Centers for Disease Control currently recommends that all people who have slept in a space with bats consider getting the rabies vaccine. Partly due to this recommendation in place since 1999, about 40,000 Americans receive the rabies shots each year.

CHANGING PATTERN OF RABIES: THE TEXAS STORY

Dogs as Initial Carriers

Texas provides an interesting case study for the spread of rabies in the new world. Although rabies was widely described in several cultures for centuries, there was no mention of rabies by the early settlers of Texas. The details of the Texas rabies story can be found at the website of the Texas Department of State Health Services (Texas Department of State Health Services, 2004). Dogs were very common among Native American tribes, but no surviving Native American folklore describes such a disease. The Spanish explorers introduced European dogs to the Americas in the 1490s. Rabies was not described in the travel memoirs of these early explorers, or the medical teams that accompanied them. Several visits by Spanish and French explorers did not note the presence of rabies in Texas through the 15th–18th centuries. The migration of pioneer settlers introduced several new diseases, such as yellow fever and smallpox, into the newly established settlements and the nearby indigenous Native American populations. The symptoms of rabies were known universally and the absence of any documentation by all of these individuals strongly suggests that rabies was not present in Texas until the 1800s.

The first references to rabid animals in Texas appear in anecdotal accounts by cowboys. These stories mention attacks by "hydrophobia cats" or "phoby cats" while sleeping on the ground in open fields. These terms were also used to describe rabid spotted skunks. Some of the stories portray the cowboys being bitten on the nose and the difficulty in getting the animal to release the bite.

Because of the rising incidence of rabies, the Texas Quarantine Act of 1856 was passed and formed the nucleus for public health acts in Texas. A state health agency called the Texas Quarantine Department was formed, which later transformed into the Texas Public Health Department. In 1903, the Pasteur Institute was opened in Austin, which produced the Pasteur vaccine for rabies prophylaxis.

Rabies in Foxes

After 1945, rabies epidemics were gradually noticed in Texas among the local gray foxes. The rapidly expanding rabies among foxes in the wild advanced up to 20 miles a month. All counties were affected eventually. Losses among farm animals were as high as $100,000 in some counties. As many as 200 persons received the rabies vaccine and treatments in several counties. A total of 1,095 cases of rabies in gray foxes were reported during a 10-year period during those times in Texas. The popularity of fox hunting worsened the situation.

The late 1940s was a watershed in rabies control in Texas and elsewhere in the United States. Veterinarians actively recommended immunization of dogs and cats and effective animal control as strategies to stop the spread of rabies to humans. Human rabies cases decreased remarkably during the 1940s and 1950s. Once rabies was controlled effectively in domestic dogs, the primary vector of rabies to humans changed from dogs to wildlife, such as skunks. In 1947, there was an epidemic of rabies in skunks in the Austin area, with 847 positive cases of rabies reported. An antirabies campaign was initiated in December to vaccinate all dogs in the area. Priority was also given to control the stray dog population. The two dog wardens impounded 6,000 animals; 35 cases of rabies were detected among these animals, 28 coming from within the city limits of Austin.

Skunk Rabies Takes Over

In 1952, wholesale killing of skunks before the cold season was advised in areas where skunk rabies was prevalent. Selective thinning of the fox population was tried in the early 1950s to control the spread of rabies in foxes. Massive vaccination drives for dogs, accompanied by an intense publicity campaign on rabies awareness, remained the focal point of rabies control. Around this time, four of the most extensive bat colonies in the United States were found in Texas: Ney Cave near Bandera, Bracken Cave in Comal County, Frio Cave in Uvalde County, and Devil's Sinkhole in Edwards County. Rabies was prevalent among vampire bats across the border in Mexico and was a threat to cattle farmers. Scientists feared that Texas bats were likely to be infected during their southern migration and would spread the disease around the state. In 1956, the first cases of rabies in bat populations were detected.

Death of a Researcher: Bat Rabies

George Menzies was a famous researcher who carried out several field investigations and published research papers on bat rabies. He contracted rabies and died in 1956. The researchers had to navigate caves harboring thousands of bats to obtain data for their studies. Mr. Menzies was most likely exposed to an aerosolized rabies virus while working in Frio Cave in Uvalde County, Texas, which is a favorite roosting cave for thousands of Mexican free-tailed bats. Mr. Menzies was said to be suffering from a poison ivy reaction as well as a possible skin infection. The abraded areas around his shoulders and neck may have facilitated the entry of the virus from the aerosols of the cave air into the body. Alternatively, a rabid bat might have bitten the researcher and the bite went unnoticed. An avian-based rabies vaccine was advised for bat researchers in the aftermath of the tragedy.

In 1959, a resurgence of fox rabies was seen in Texas. Skunk rabies was also common. In contrast, rabies in raccoon and bobcats was relatively rare. A skunk rabies epizootic began in the 1970s that peaked in 1979 and lasted until 1985. An epizootic is a pattern of disease in which large numbers of animals are affected at the same time. During this particular rabies epizootic, 5,070 cases of rabies in skunks were reported. Periodic outbreaks of canine rabies were also noted throughout the 1970s in Texas.

In 1987, an epizootic of rabies among the gray foxes was noted in the western parts of the state. Spillover cases of rabies were also noted in raccoons, cats, bobcats, goats, and cattle. In 1988, a rabies epizootic in coyotes was noted in the southern parts of the state. The molecular analysis of the virus proved that it was derived from the domestic canine rabies variety from Mexico. This coyote epizootic also spread to unvaccinated domestic dogs.

Oral Rabies Vaccine Program for Wildlife

In 1994, state agencies took up an oral rabies vaccination program in Texas to prevent rabies in wild animals. The Texas Department of Health partnered with the Ontario (Canada) Ministry of Natural Resources that had several initiatives in the control of rabies in wild animals. The aim of this program was to create a barrier to the spread of the rabies in the wild by forming a band of immune animals. There were two ongoing rabies epizootics in the state at that time: one caused by the domestic dog/coyote variant in south Texas, and another caused by the gray fox variant in west/central Texas. Initially, studies were done among coyotes to find out the ideal method to deliver the vaccine. Flavored bait for coyotes was chosen as the preferred method. The first field trials of the oral rabies vaccine for coyotes were conducted in south Texas. Vaccine-laden baits were distributed on an annual basis every winter. The baiting strategy successfully eliminated the virus from Texas.

In 1996, field trials of oral rabies vaccine for gray foxes were conducted in west/central Texas. Vaccine-laden baits were distributed on an annual basis every winter. This program successfully stopped the expansion of the rabies epizootic in foxes in Texas.

The saga of control of wild rabies in Texas is a triumph of public health measures. The coordinated work of several departments, the dedication of a host of individuals and researchers, epitomized by George Menzies who tragically died of rabies, is an example of how this disease can be controlled.

Currently rabies is seen in several parts of the world. Only some of the island nations are considered rabies-free. Several developing nations are a hot bed for rabies because of poor domestic and wildlife animal control programs, the high prevalence of stray animals, and lack of funds. The human cost of rabies all over the world is enormous. Most of the cases are reported from poor developing nations without the infrastructure to monitor and employ preventative programs to stop transmission among the dog, the most common carrier. Stray dogs constitute an important mode of transmission of rabies in different parts of the world. By World Health Organization estimates, at least 55,000 people die worldwide every year because of rabies. There are very few survivors of the disease once the individual develops signs of the infection. This figure of 55,000 deaths is probably a vast underestimation, with the actual number of rabies deaths much higher because of the lack of proper reporting systems. Although the incidence of rabies is not high in the developed world, the economic costs are high because of the expense of postexposure prophylaxis and the cost to control the spread of sylvatic rabies among wild animals.

2

How One Gets Infected with Rabies

STRAY KITTEN FOUND BY A FAMILY ON THE WAY BACK HOME

A family returning from a vacation stopped at a fast food restaurant in south central Texas, where the two daughters were approached by an especially friendly kitten. The kitten was thin, alert, and obviously homeless. The girls succeeded in persuading their parents to adopt the kitten. On returning home, the family took the kitten to a veterinarian for vaccinations and de-worming. The veterinarian thought the kitten was approximately four months old and in good health. A taeniafuge (an agent or medicine for expelling tapeworms from the body) was administered, and the kitten was vaccinated against usual infections of cats. Inactivated rabies vaccine was also given intramuscularly in a hind limb. The kitten was subdued for the rest of the day. The kitten could not be found the next day and later it was discovered to be hiding in a closet. The kitten seemed apprehensive and tried to escape and hide. It was not eating or drinking water.

The kitten was returned to the veterinary clinic on the third day. It was agitated and showed extreme nervousness and slight weakness of the hind legs. The veterinarian left the kitten after the examination. When she came back towards the cat it attacked violently, inflicting several bites and scratches to

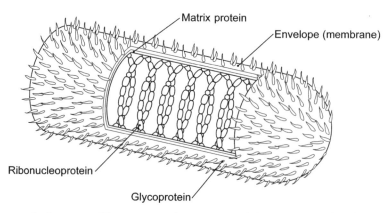

Structure of rabies virus. The outer envelope consists of glycoprotein with spike-like projections. The inner core consist of single stranded ribonucleic acid (RNA) that forms ribonucleoprotein in combination with nucleocapsid proteins. (Drawn by Jeff Dixon)

the veterinarian and a veterinary assistant. Although the locality was essentially a rabies-free area, the kitten was euthanatized, and the head was submitted to the Texas Department of Health Laboratory. Rabies was confirmed by immunofluorescence test. Subsequent testing revealed that the rabies viral strain was probably of skunk origin (Clark, 1988).

The family was advised to seek the advice of a physician regarding postexposure prophylaxis. Both the veterinarian and the veterinary assistant, each of whom had received pre-exposure rabies vaccinations before, were given two doses each of human diploid cell rabies vaccine, with an interval of 3 days between doses.

This case illustrates a typical scenario in which an unvaccinated stray animal is adopted or comes in close contact with children or adults. The behavioral changes in the kitten should evoke the suspicion of rabies. Classically rabies is associated with the bites of rabid dogs. The pattern is changing in the United States, with several wild animals posing the threat of rabies transmission. Since 1946, ten cases of human rabies have been associated with bites of rabid or suspected rabid cats.

STRUCTURE OF THE RABIES VIRUS

Viral particles of rabies were first observed by Matsumoto from Kyoto, Japan (Matsumoto, 1963). Rabies virus is approximately 180 nm long and 75 nm wide. The structure resembles a bullet. The core is made up of helical ribonucleoprotein where the genome is coded. The outer glycoprotein envelope has several spike-like projections. The center of the virion is made up of single-stranded genomic RNA (ribonucleic acid) that is bound to the nucleocapsid protein, forming a RNP (ribonucleoprotein) complex. The RNP is in the form of a helical structure. This is not to be confused with the helical structure of the DNA seen in some viruses and several higher animals such as human beings. Unlike the RNA, DNA is double stranded. Two other proteins, L (Large) and P (phosphorylation) proteins, also exist within the virion. The L and P proteins have important roles in the replication of the virus. L protein is a viral RNA-dependent RNA polymerase. This enzyme helps to form new virions from the parent virus with the help of the host cellular machinery. The envelope of the virus consists of G (surface) proteins. The part of the membrane of the host cell from which the virus was formed through budding is also contained in the envelope. It is almost as if the virus tore off part of the host cell membrane to form a coat for itself on the way out! The other protein, M (matrix) protein, covers the inner wall of the envelope.

Multiplication of Rabies Virus

The rabies virus cannot live or replicate by itself. It needs a host cell to perform this function and propagate. It acts intelligently in a Trojan-horse fashion in this regard. The fusion of the rabies virus envelope to the host cell membrane indicates infection. The virus penetrates the cell membrane, enters the cytoplasm, and aggregates in the large endosomes. The viral membranes fuse to the endosomes. This results in the release of the viral genetic material into the cytoplasm. A viral polymerase enzyme uses the cell's resources to manufacture an RNA strand. Simultaneously, the cellular powerhouses of the endoplasmic reticulum and Golgi bodies are used by the virus in this process of synthesizing various viral proteins. The new RNA strand processed in the cell is encapsulated by the various new proteins. The new viral particle migrates towards the cell surface and is coated by the plasma membrane, and the nascent viral particle buds from the plasma membrane.

The structure and method of replication of this tiny virus is so well coordinated to ensure the continued propagation of the virus in the host once it infects the cell. The genes controlling the production of various proteins are encoded in the central RNA strip. As this complicated process of replication unravels, each gene produces the corresponding protein. As in an orchestra, everything falls into its respective position, forming a nascent virion. The budding of the young virion through the host cell membrane causes the destruction of the host cell. Thousands of virions escape and start infecting other healthy cells. The disease advances with progressive involvement of more and more cells. This vicious cycle goes on, infecting more and more host cells, until the animal becomes severely affected.

The method of reproduction of viruses is unique in nature because it uses the cellular machinery of another organism. Experts debate whether viruses are living objects in the strictest sense but agree that they can cause havoc, especially because of their small size. This also makes them extremely difficult to detect. We do not have simple tests to detect viruses yet. Culturing viruses is difficult, requiring unique media, and is only done in specialized laboratories.

ANIMALS IMPORTANT IN RABIES TRANSMISSION

Domestic Dogs

The most common vector of rabies all over the world is the domestic dog. In developed countries, the incidence of rabies transmitted by dogs is almost zero because of excellent dog rabies vaccination programs. Interestingly, in the United States the most common vector of the disease is bats. The incidence of rabies in the United States has come down from the 70 or so cases per year several years ago to one or two cases per year during the past few decades. The pathogenesis in animals is complicated; generally the animal is infected by a carrier or an infected animal from the wild. There are some similarities of infection in animals and humans. Generally the virus travels along the nerve fibers to the spinal cord and the brain of the animals. This propensity of the viruses to zoom into neural tissue is called (or known as) neurotropism.

Rabies has a short incubation period in dogs, usually 14–60 days. This is the interval between the entry of the virus into the animal's body and the manifestation of the disease. This indicates the time taken by the virus to travel to the brain from the site of the bite. The animals can have a prodromal phase in which they exhibit features like anorexia, fever, and restlessness in the beginning of the illness. The area of the skin where the virus has entered might become hypersensitive because of the involvement of the sensory nerves. The animals might exhibit behavior of increased rubbing or even mutilating behavior towards those body parts because of the irritation. Within a few days the virus goes through the nerves, gets into the spinal cord, and subsequently travels up towards the brain. In the brain, the viruses can infect any cell and cause inflammation; this is called an encephalomyelitis. The functions of every neuronal cell can be severely impaired. The animal exhibits impaired affect, confusion, and aggressive behaviors. They can be highly excitable and show increased startle reflexes. They become aggressive. They can bite or

attack animate or inanimate objects unprovoked, and these bites can be ferocious. The animal might cling to the person bitten without releasing its hold
on the victim. These bites are dangerous because by this time the rabies virus
is teeming in the brain and has started its journey down the cranial nerves.
Cranial nerves are the large nerves directly originating from the brain and
connect to structures in the head and neck, for which they carry out important
functions. Importantly, nerves coming from the brain also supply the salivary
glands. This offers a route for the virus to travel from the brain and settle in
the salivary gland. Thus a high concentration of the virus is achieved in the
saliva and the biting animal is able to transmit the disease through the saliva.
Several muscles of the face can go into spasms. The jaw can droop and paralysis of several muscles of the face can set in. The animal is unable to bark, but
may howl in high-pitched tones. It cannot even swallow its own saliva and
drools excessively. There is paralysis of the muscles of the neck and the animal
cannot eat or drink. It becomes weak and dehydrated (Jackson and Wunner,
2002, 169). The drooling saliva can be thick and slimy, teaming with millions
of the virus particles. Ultimately the animal cannot move because a spreading
paralysis takes over the whole body.

Various species of animals can have some variation of this general illness. In
the case of dogs, younger dogs may be more susceptible to rabies. There are
believed to be two types of rabies in general: furious rabies and dumb rabies.
The furious rabies is more common. The animal can be more active and potentially dangerous, inflicting bites on unsuspecting individuals. In furious rabies,
the animal can be predominantly agitated and aggressive. The dumb variety is
characterized by weakness and paralysis. These two types of rabies may indicate
the level of viral infection in different parts of the brain. Even in furious rabies,
the animal can become paralyzed towards the end stages of the disease. This is
not to be confused with paralytic rabies. Both types of the disease have distinct
features and the exact reason why these two disease forms exist is unknown.
The classical features of human rabies, namely hydrophobia (fear of water) and
aerophobia (fear of air), are not usually seen in animal rabies. As the disease
progresses, the animal can also exhibit seizures and autonomic system hyperac-
tivity in the form of hyperventilation, hypertension, tremors, and uncontrolled
body temperatures (both high and low). Ultimately, irregular cardiac rhythm
can set in. The animal will develop cardiac and respiratory arrest and slip into
a coma. Death can occur from any number of conditions as mentioned earlier
or from a combination of events.

The practice of quarantine in many animals, mainly dogs, has been derived
from field observations. The standard practice is a 6-month quarantine if an animal is bitten by a suspected wild animal carrying rabies. By that time almost any

animal that will develop rabies should do so. The reports of chronic rabies carriers in several animal species are not substantiated. The usual practice of quarantine after a dog bites a person is to observe the animal for 10 days. This is because by day ten the animal should show profound features of the infection. If the animal dies during this time, the diagnosis of rabies can be confirmed by a postmortem examination of the animal. One of the useful confirmatory features is Negri bodies, which can be found microscopically in the brain. Recently, salivary tests for the rabies virus antigen in dog saliva have been developed. These tests were noted to have a high sensitivity and specificity. The potential shortfall of this method is the possibility of intermittent shedding of the virus by the infected animal and hence a diagnosis can be missed.

Cats

Cats outnumber dogs in the United States as the most common domestic animal. Naturally, in the United States, the cat is the foremost domestic animal diagnosed with rabies. Between 1991 and 1998 there were 2,173 cases of rabies in domestic cats with an average of 272 cases reported yearly nationwide. There are several reasons for this preponderance. Apart from being the largest animal population, the vaccination rates for rabies in cats is lower than dogs. Public awareness regarding the potential for cats to get infected with rabies may be low. Cats are also nocturnal and many roam around unsupervised and expose themselves to attacks with rabies-infected wild animals such as raccoons or skunks. Cats are also curious creatures and their examining behavior with small animals also might place them in jeopardy. In the United States, cats are likely to be infected by a raccoon on the East Coast from Florida to Maine and by a skunk in the Midwest and California. Bats are also another source of infection to cats. The origin of the infecting virus can be pinpointed with relative accuracy because there are several variants of the virus in nature. The viruses in skunk and raccoon vary. This variation can be determined by performing a genetic analysis of the virus. Geographical variation of the viruses is also noted among isolates from different regions of the country.

Cat rabies usually amounts to less than 0.1 percent of dog rabies all over the world. In the United States more cats are diagnosed to have rabies because of the dramatic decrease in the incidence of dog rabies by preventive efforts. Cat rabies in the United States usually occurs in unvaccinated animals and of younger (less than 1 year) age. Cats may be more prone for spillover infection from bats than dogs.

Rabies associated with cats also has important public health consequences. An investigation in 2007 spanning several states attests to this (CDC, 2008d).

The South Atlantic Summer Showdown softball tournament was held at a recreational complex in Spartanburg County, South Carolina, from July 13 to 15, 2007. One of the coaches found an apparently healthy kitten in a garbage can and adopted it. The kitten was placed in a box and brought to several games. Two days later, the kitten was behaving abnormally and was taken to a veterinarian. The veterinarian found the kitten to be severely ill and the kitten was euthanized. Rabies was not suspected initially, but later, because of a mother's insistence, testing was done and the kitten was found to be positive for rabies.

A multi-state epidemiological investigation ensued and several persons who had contact with the kitten during the tournament were identified. Thirty-eight of the 60 teams that participated reported at least one person exposed to the rabid kitten. Of these, 27 persons were identified and offered postexposure prophylaxis: 1 from South Carolina, 15 from Georgia, 11 from North Carolina, and none from Tennessee. All of them had actual exposure to the kitten's saliva, either through a bite, a lick on the oral or nasal mucosa, or a claw scratch.

Cattle

Livestock can also be affected with rabies. This is more commonly reported in areas such as Latin America. Bats are the predominant source of their infection. In the United States, raccoons and skunks can also infect cattle. Infected cattle exhibit similar behavior to dogs. They can go through a prodromal phase culminating in severe paralysis and death. Horses and sheep can also be infected similarly and have a similar fate. These animals could also pose a danger to the public during exhibits and carnivals. Multiple rabies exposures have occurred, requiring extensive public health investigation and medical follow-up. For example, thousands of persons received rabies postexposure prophylaxis after being exposed to rabid or potentially rabid animal species (including cats, goats, bears, sheep, ponies, and dogs) at a pet store in New Hampshire, a county fair in New York State, petting zoos in Iowa and Texas, and during school and rodeo events in Wyoming. Although no rabies deaths have been reported under these circumstances, the Centers for Disease Control and Prevention (CDC) states that these situations create substantial public health and medical care challenges, such as tracking down the exposed individuals and providing postexposure prophylaxis.

Rabies in Goats

A goat that was shown at a county fair in New York State in 1996 developed rabies (Chang, 2002). Approximately 25,000 people attended the fair. Out of these, 2,700 individuals were evaluated for potential exposure to the rabid goat; 465 of them were treated with rabies vaccine for rabies exposure at a cost of half a million dollars. Some states and counties do require that any animal being shown in fairs must be vaccinated against rabies and hold a valid certificate. There are no approved vaccines for rabies in several animals, goats being a prime example. Vaccine manufacturers did not have any incentive to develop specific vaccines for these animals because of the small market. Off-label use of rabies vaccines licensed in other animals is permitted in these circumstances although their exact efficacy is unknown. A licensed veterinarian should be consulted for proper advice.

Foxes

Foxes are part of the canine family. Foxes and wolves can become infected in the wild, acting as prominent carriers of the infection to the urban cycle. Foxes can also be affected by viruses such as canine distemper virus and the clinical manifestations can closely resemble that of rabies. In the middle to late 1700s, fox and dog rabies was very common in the former British colonies throughout the world. Part of reason was the enthusiasm for fox hunting and probable importation of animals into newly acquired territories. In Canada the Governor General was bitten by a pet fox and died of rabies in 1819. Fox rabies is prevalent worldwide. In the United States, fox rabies is identified in the East Coast and the Southwest. Any fox should be handled carefully. A wild fox should never be touched or approached. Signs of rabies in foxes include having no fear of humans, acting aggressively, or acting listless. Any suspicious animal should be reported to the local animal control officer.

Raccoons

Raccoons have evolved into one of the most important rabies reservoir in the continental United States. They are highly adaptable and have a high density of population in the wild. The original source of raccoon rabies was suspected in Florida in the 1940s. Although not proven, it is now widely believed that during the next 30 years the raccoon rabies spread north along the Atlantic coast, infecting several states. The spread of the infection is geographically prevented by the Appalachian Mountains to some extent. Even with detailed studies, the exact nature of the illness in raccoons is not known. There is a wide variety of susceptibilities and the infected animals may also lack the clinical features previously described that are common in other wildlife species. Raccoons can also be affected by canine distemper virus, closely mimicking rabies, with a high mortality rate. Canine distemper is a highly contagious disease of wild and domestic carnivores. This is caused by a virus that infects animals such as the gray fox, raccoons, coyotes, skunks, and weasels. Although related to measles virus, canine distemper virus poses no known threat to humans. A vaccine is available to protect domestic pets from this disease. In the wild, this disease is most prevalent in raccoons in the southeastern United States and has wiped out several raccoon populations.

Skunks

Interestingly, skunks are the most important reservoir of rabies everywhere in the United States except the East Coast. Infection in skunks could have spread by the western exploration of the country in the 1800s. Rabid skunks can be ferocious biters. The clinical features of the disease can be hard to detect in skunks as in any other wild animal. For this reason skunks are not ideal animals to be kept as pets. Infected skunks can exhibit abnormal behaviors such as being active during daylight hours, appearing to have no fear of humans or animals, being easy to approach, acting aggressively, or acting listless or sick. Contact of domestic pets with skunks should be limited and a local animal control agency should be appraised of any suspicious animals.

Coyotes

The coyote is one of the best runners in the canine family. They can run up to 40 miles per hour and can jump as high as 14 feet. Coyotes are another possible reservoir of rabies, but for unknown reasons they do not play an important role in the propagation of rabies in any part of the world, including the United States. Sporadic cases are reported including two human cases reported in association with a coyote rabies outbreak in Texas in 1991 and 1994. The features of rabies in coyotes could be wandering during daytime, acting aggressively without any fear of humans, and acting listless. As with all wild animals, one should never touch or approach a coyote. Although the incidence of rabies is low in coyotes compared with other wild animals, any coyote should be treated as potentially capable of spreading the infection.

BATS AND RABIES

Bats are an important reservoir of rabies worldwide. The southern United States and Mexico have some of the largest bat colonies in the world. However, in some cases the current bat populations are only a fraction of those thought to have been present in the recent past. *Tadarida brasiliensis* (the Mexican free-tailed bat) forms the largest known mammalian aggregations, with colonies in Texas currently reaching 20 million bats (McCracken, 1986) in a single cave. However, at some known roost caves, populations declined in the 1950s and 1960s by as much as 99 percent. During the beginning of this century, domestic dogs caused the highest number of cases of human rabies. This has become progressively rare and other animals have taken the place of the dog. About 236 human rabies infections were reported in the United States from 1946 to 1965. From 1946 through 1949, the number of human rabies infections averaged 24 per year, declining to 1.5 per year from 1962 through 1965. Ninety percent of rabies cases were caused by dog bites from 1946 through 1949, decreasing to 67 percent from 1962 through 1965. From 1970 to 1989, only 45 percent of rabies cases were caused by canine rabies virus variants (all but one was acquired outside of the United States), 30 percent were caused by bat rabies variants, and one was caused by a corneal transplant from an unsuspected rabies patient. From 1990 through 2000, bat rabies virus variants have emerged as the predominant cause of human rabies in the United States. Thirty-two deaths occurred during this period, and 24 (75 percent) were due to bat rabies virus.

The most vexing problem with bat rabies is that only 2 (8 percent) of the 24 patients with human rabies caused by bat rabies virus gave a definitive history of a bat bite. Nine patients (38 percent) had a history of direct physical contact with bats, five (21 percent) had a history of a bat inside the living area, and eight (33 percent) had no history of proximity to bats. Rabies has also been reported in several instances when people have spent prolonged periods in bat-infested caves. This could be due to the contact with aerosolized rabies virus particles that might be present in bat-infested caves. Alternatively, bats could inflict bites in the dark conditions of a cave and one might not notice. One reason why bat bites may be unnoticed is that bats usually inflict relatively smaller bites because of the smaller size of their teeth in contrast to other carnivorous mammals such as dogs. Bat bites also do not tend to draw any blood. Furthermore, public awareness about the rabies potential of bat bites or contact may be low.

Bat Rabies in Connecticut, 1995

A 13-year-old girl from Greenwich, Connecticut, reported general fatigue, stiffness, tremors, and tingling in her left arm and hand on September 18, 1995. On September 22, she presented to the local emergency room (CDC, 1996). She had a low-grade fever. Cervical radiculopathy was presumptively diagnosed and was attributed to her habit of carrying a heavy backpack; ibuprofen (a pain killer) was prescribed. Cervical radiculopathy involves the nerves coming out of the spinal cord at the neck region and can cause pain radiating from the neck to the arms. The patient was given a cervical collar and referred to a pediatric neurologist.

Three days later, on September 25, her symptoms persisted and the doctor noted sensory changes on the left arm and face. She was admitted to a hospital the same day. She had a fever (temperature was 100°F). She was alert but anxious; rigidity upon moving the neck was noted by the physicians. Blood test results indicated a white blood cell (WBC) count of 13,600/μL (normal is 5,000–10,000/μL). Her cerebrospinal fluid (CSF) showed 100 white cells/μL (normal is 0–5/μL) and slightly elevated protein of 104 mg/dL (normal is less than 40 mg/dL). These findings are potentially indicative of an inflammation of the coverings of the brain known as meningitis. Meningitis can occur independently or in combination with an inflammation of the brain (meningoencephalitis).

The possibility of a meningoencephalitis was suspected in this case. Lyme disease is common in the northeast and it can produce a meningoencephalitis. Because of this suspicion, intravenous antibiotics and steroids were administered to counter Lyme disease. She became intermittently drowsy and agitated. She was occasionally disoriented in the 24 hours after admission. Subsequently, the tongue deviated to the right (indicating paralysis of the nerve supplying the tongue muscles), unequal sized pupils (indicating paralysis of some of the nerves supplying the tiny muscles of the iris of the eye) developed, and progressive weakness of the left arm was also noted. She was apprehensive and had difficulty swallowing, accompanied by a prominent aversion to oral intake. Severe pharyngeal spasms were elicited by offering a drink of water. The diagnosis of rabies was considered, and the patient was placed in isolation. She became increasingly agitated and hallucinated. She was intermittently lucid and self-reflective and apologized for her mood and hallucinations.

On September 26, the girl was transferred to the intensive-care unit, where she was placed on a respirator because of concerns of respiratory failure. She became progressively less responsive the next day and subsequently lapsed into a coma. Rabies was diagnosed on October 2 at the New York State Rabies Laboratory on the basis of corneal impressions of the patient collected on October 1, which were positive for rabies virus by immunofluorescence technique. Rabies virus tests done on the blood were also positive. Rising titers of rabies virus neutralizing antibody of 1:32, 1:64, and 1:512 in three serum samples collected on September 25, 29, and October 2, respectively, were noted. The diagnosis was confirmed at the CDC through the extraction of viral nucleic acid from the saliva and corneal epithelia. The virus material was reverse-transcribed with rabies-specific primers and amplified using the polymerase chain reaction (PCR) assay. Final testing at CDC, including the specific nucleotide sequencing of the final PCR products, characterized the rabies virus as a variant associated with the silver-haired bat, *Lasionycterus noctivagans.*

Despite intensive treatment, her condition did not improve. On October 3, mechanical ventilation was withdrawn, and the patient died. This was the first case of human rabies reported in Connecticut since 1932.

The girl lived in a single-family dwelling in a wooded residential area in Greenwich, Connecticut. Although she denied a history of animal bites, multiple potential sources of animal contact were present in the home and surrounding environment. All domestic animals with which she was known to have had contact were accounted for and were found to be well, without any signs of rabies. Following the diagnosis of rabies, the girl's family recalled that on approximately August 19, almost a month before she became symptomatic, a bat flying inside the house struck at least one person. The girl was asleep in an upstairs bedroom at that time. Inspection of the house and surrounding property by the Greenwich Department of Health on September 29 did not identify any dead animals or evidence of bats. Because of possible percutaneous or mucous membrane contact with the girl's secretions between September 10 and October 3, rabies postexposure prophylaxis was administered to 83 persons who reported probable contact with the patient's saliva: 46 health-care workers, 29 children, four family members, three family friends intimately involved in the girl's care, and one other adult. This case illustrates the usual lack of clear-cut history of bat bites in bat-virus-associated rabies. The bite might have been too trivial to be noticed. In such cases in which a bat is found in the bedroom, it may be prudent to obtain postexposure prophylaxis for rabies because the person may never know if the bat has bitten them while they were sleeping.

Bat Rabies in California, 2003

A previously healthy 66-year-old man who lived in Trinity County, California, was admitted to a hospital emergency department in September 2003 with complaints of chest pain (CDC, 2003). In the beginning, he had drowsiness, headache, and malaise for 2 weeks followed by right arm pain and paresthesias, and a 1-day history of right-hand weakness. The arm pain was sharp and severe. The patient reported being bitten by a bat on the right index finger while in his bed approximately 5 weeks before admission. He removed the bat from his home, and it flew away. The patient washed the wound but did not seek any postexposure prophylaxis for rabies. Rabies was suspected in the emergency room and treatment was promptly started in the emergency room. He received a rabies vaccine, rabies immune globulin, ribavirin (an antiviral drug), and interferon-alpha on the day of admission followed by a second dose of rabies vaccine 3 days later. The vaccine was given in the hope of stimulating any antibody response since it is usually too late to give the vaccine if a patient has signs and symptoms of the disease.

On admission, he was afebrile, alert, and oriented. He had decreased right upper extremity strength, decreased sensation to light touch, and slight impairment in his ability to concentrate. His WBC count was elevated at 13,900 cells/μL (normal is 3,700–9,400 cells/μL). All other laboratory values were within the normal range.

While in the hospital, the patient had steady neurological decline during the following week. Progressive confusion and disorientation ensued. He developed a fever and on the fourth hospital day an artificial breathing machine was used for airway protection. He was in a coma. By the fifth hospital day, an X-ray of the chest was abnormal. His electroencephalogram (brain wave mapping) showed diffuse slowing. He died from rabies on September 14, 2003, approximately 6 weeks after being bitten by a bat.

Bat Rabies in Mississippi, 2005

On September 11, 2005, a 10-year-old boy complained of fever and headache. A pediatrician saw him on September 13 and diagnosed a viral illness. Fever persisted and the boy was taken to the emergency room on September 15. All tests including blood tests and X-rays were normal and he was discharged home.

His condition worsened throughout the day with fever, progressive paresthesias of the right side of the scalp and right arm, dysphagia, disorientation, and ataxia. The same evening he developed fever, insomnia, and urinary urgency. He returned to the emergency room and was admitted with a diagnosis of encephalitis. The tests upon admission showed slightly elevated white cell count and slight increase in protein in the CSF, obtained through a spinal tap.

His condition deteriorated rapidly after admission. Speech became slurred, and he began to hallucinate. He became increasingly agitated and combative and required sedation. In his agitated state, the patient bit a family member. The next morning the patient was transferred to a tertiary care facility. Within hours after transfer, he became lethargic and was put on a respirator. Tests for common infections that affect the brain such as West Nile, St. Louis, Rocky Mountain spotted fever, Herpes simplex virus, and enterovirus infections were negative. His condition worsened during the next 10 days. He remained on the respirator with wide fluctuations in blood pressure and temperature. Because of massive swelling of the brain, brain herniation occurred. Life support was withdrawn, and the patient died on September 27.

This case was referred to CDC's Unexplained Deaths and Critical Illness Project (UNEX) for additional diagnostic testing (CDC, 2005). Doctors suspected rabies because of the rapidly progressive nature of the disease. On October 5, CDC diagnosed rabies on the basis of blood tests that indicated an increase in rabies virus specific IgG antibody titer from 128 to 8,192 in paired serum samples collected on September 16 and 21. Subsequent testing of CSF demonstrated the presence of rabies-virus-specific antibodies.

This patient did not have any definite history of contact with an animal with rabies risk. However, after the child's death, several persons reported that bats were commonly seen outside the home. On two occasions, dead bats were also discovered inside the home and an attached garage. A live bat was caught in an apartment above the garage during the summer of 2005. The child had removed a live bat from his bedroom and released it outdoors in the spring of 2005.

The child had also attended a summer camp in Alabama for several weeks in July. The participants stayed overnight in a nearby cavern used for tours and special events. There was no indication of direct contact with bats at the camp or in the cavern, although one bat was reportedly observed clinging to the rocky wall inside the cavern.

The investigators concluded that the exposure to bats at the boy's home was the likely source of rabies. The findings underscore the importance of recognizing the risk for rabies from direct contact with bats and seeking prompt medical attention when exposure occurs.

These cases illustrate the potential danger of rabies with exposure to bats in the United States. Although not common, such an eventuality could be prevented if proper precautions are carried out. Messages to the public should emphasize that bats can transmit rabies virus to humans. Bats should never be kept as pets. Bats should be excluded from human living quarters and should never be handled with bare hands. When a bat is found in living quarters and the possibility exists that an unrecognized exposure has occurred, the animal should be submitted to a local public health laboratory for diagnostic testing. If tests are positive for rabies virus, proper postexposure prophylaxis should be given to all of the contacts of the index case. On the contrary, if the tests are negative, there are no grounds for concern and unnecessary prophylaxis given to contacts could be avoided.

Vampire Bats

The world has more than 900 species of bats, and only three species are vampire bats. These bats are exclusive to the Americas and important in the spread of rabies in Latin America. All three species of vampire bats occur in Latin America. Contrary to the popular myth of blood-sucking vampires, the

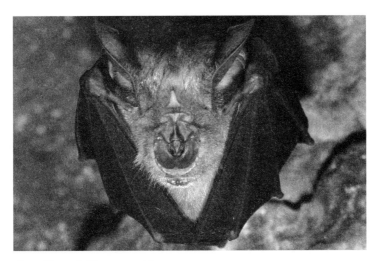

Vampire bat. (Demark/Shutterstock)

vampire bats do not like the taste of human blood and have only done this in rare instances. *Desmodus rotundus*, the common vampire bat, is the most common and widespread species. This bat is native to east and west Mexico, Central America, and much of South America to Uruguay, northern Argentina, and central Chile. Fossil evidence indicates that vampire bats have been in the Americas since the Pleistocene period, approximately 2.5 million years ago. Vampire bat is a term used exclusively to refer to bats that feed on blood, otherwise known as hematophagus. The name "vampire" is of Slavonic origin, referring to a ghost that supposedly sucked blood from its victims.

Animal blood is the only food ingested by the vampire bat. Cattle, pigs, and horses are common victims of this bat. The sharp incisor teeth of the bat cut the skin of the victims. Two channels on each side of the bottom of the tongue permit the bat to draw the blood from the animal. The saliva of vampire bats contains a substance, draculin, which prevents the victim's blood from clotting. These bats are capable of biting any part of the body of cattle. The bites, however, are more common on the neck, ears, and around the base of the tail. A typical vampire bat can feed on up to 1 ounce of blood (30 mL) in a feeding session lasting for 20 minutes. The feeding pattern of the vampire bats has been studied by DNA analysis of the blood taken from the intestinal tract of the bats. The vampire bats are found in a variety of habitats: caves, house roofs, abandoned mines, tunnels, hollow trees, wells, and so forth. The bats usually form stable colonies and the individual population of the colonies differs widely. The average number of bats could be between 10 and 300. The number of individuals in a colony appears to depend on the availability of food, space, and suitable climatic conditions. Large colonies have more than 2,000 animals. At roosting times, especially in the evening, they can be seen forming a cloud of flying creatures in the evening sky. Interestingly, moonlight influences the foraging behavior of the vampire bat. No vampire activity is seen on moonlit nights.

Vampire-bat-transmitted rabies has probably existed in tropical America even before the European explorations. Fernandez de Oviedo, in his book, *Sumario de la Historia Natural de las Indias*, mentioned that many soldiers died from bat bites during the Darien conquest in the early 16th century, and Molina Solis, in *Historia del Descubrimiento y Conquista de Yucatán*, mentioned that many soldiers and horses of Francesco de Montejo's army were attacked by vampire bats.

The first report concerning bovine rabies in tropical America was made by Carini in 1911, from São Paulo, Brazil. He observed Negri bodies in a bovine brain in postmortem examination of the cattle. Negri bodies are the telltale sign of rabies infection seen in the infected brain under the microscope; the visualization of this abnormality is virtually pathognomonic of rabies. He was also able to produce paralytic rabies in rabbits by injecting them with this material. Pawan first isolated the rabies virus in 1931 from different species of bats. "Derringue," a fatal paralytic disease of cattle seen in Mexico, was proven to be caused by the rabies virus. Years later, paralytic bovine rabies caused by vampire bats has been described in Venezuela, Central America, and Panama. This variety of animal rabies is only seen in the Americas in areas 1,800–2,000 m above sea level and at latitudes between 33°S and 28°N. The important limiting factor for vampire bats is winter temperature; they cannot live in areas where the temperature drops below 15°C.

OTHER ANIMALS

More than 50 percent of all rabies cases in the United States involve raccoons. Skunks (22.5 percent), foxes (6.5 percent), and insectivorous bats (10 percent) are other common carriers. Rabies is also rarely found in smaller mammals such as rabbits, squirrels, rats, and opossums. Domestic animals account for less than 10 percent of all rabies cases in the United States.

Rarely, other wild animals can also be the carriers of rabies. Despite the abundant population of different rodents, documented cases of rabies are uncommon in these animal species. No reservoir for rabies is identified in rodents so far. Rabies in beavers has been documented, with some bizarre behavior shown by the animals. In June 1997, a beaver in Chatham County,

Jordan Lake in Canada, swam towards a boat and tried to jump into the boat and attack the fishermen. It was killed with a paddle. In August 1997, another beaver was spotted in the same lake and swam into a public swimming area. It bit a teenager in the arm. The animal was scared away but returned to attack other swimmers. The animal was finally pursued and killed. Rabies virus testing was positive in both the animals. Monkeys can also transmit rabies to humans in areas such as south Asia, including the Indian subcontinent and Nepal. The travel medicine center in Nepal advises that people seek medical attention for possible postexposure prophylaxis for rabies after contact (a wound, a bite, or a scratch) with any animals including monkeys. In Nepal, most animal exposures to travelers occur in Kathmandu and in a study, monkey bites or scratches accounted for 43 percent of all exposures in tourists (CIWEC Clinic Travel Medicine Center, 2007).

Horses can also become infected with rabies. Both the dumb and furious forms can be seen in horses. Behavioral characteristics are the most common sign exhibited. The animal can become aggressive towards itself or other animals and people. Self-mutilation is a characteristic feature. The animals can salivate excessively. Rabies can be misdiagnosed as colic in horses because of excessive rolling, pawing, and sweating. Other features suggestive of rabies are fever, lack of appetite, lameness, facial nerve paralysis, weakness, and restlessness progressing to lack of coordination, self-mutilation, aggressiveness, vocalization, drooling, and paralysis. If rabies is suspected, horses should be handled carefully. Direct contact with the horse should be avoided. Personnel should be double gloved if the horse is touched for the euthanasia procedure. It is preferable for such personnel to have pre-exposure prophylaxis and demonstrable high rabies antibody titers indicating immunity to rabies.

In a rabies outbreak in Zimbabwe, Africa, from 1980 to 1983, the majority of the documented animal cases occurred in jackals (74.3 percent of 404 cases). Since 1956, golden jackals (*Canis aureus*) have been one of the primary vectors maintaining endemic wildlife rabies in Israel. The mongoose acts as an important reservoir of rabies in Asia, Africa, and the Caribbean islands. Wolves are also important in rabies transmission in Asia and Africa. In 2004, a brown bear attacked and killed two men and injured six others in central Romania. The animal attacked people picking mushrooms and fell on others in another part of the woods. Hunters shot and killed the bear several hours after the attack. Tests conducted on the bear confirmed rabies.

Another unusual case of rabies was reported in 1986 in a javelina, a small piglike animal, in the state of Arizona. A 47-year-old woman and her husband were hunting for javelina near Superstition Mountains, east of Phoenix. The woman observed an animal chasing its tail. The animal became violent and bit her on the left upper thigh, and her husband had to shoot the animal to dislodge it. The animal was diagnosed to have rabies through direct immuno-fluorescent technique of the brain. The woman was given wound treatment and postexposure prophylaxis for rabies.

Rabies in Michigan: Case Study of Changing Animal Vectors

Rabies can be prevalent in a wide variety of wild carnivores in a given area. The state of Michigan is a perfect example of how rabies epidemiology has changed over the last half century in the United States. Generally, the incidence of rabies in domestic animals has decreased dramatically over the last 60 years in the United States because of intense rabies control programs. In the 1930s, there were several human cases of rabies reported per year in the

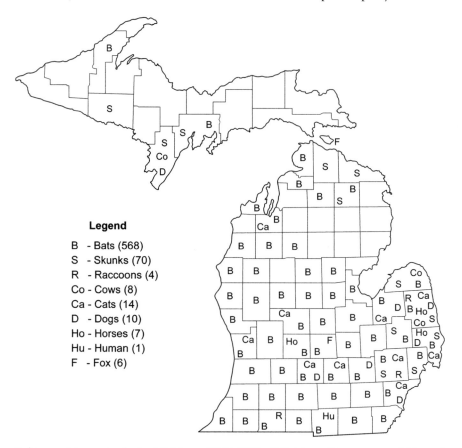

Legend

B - Bats (568)
S - Skunks (70)
R - Raccoons (4)
Co - Cows (8)
Ca - Cats (14)
D - Dogs (10)
Ho - Horses (7)
Hu - Human (1)
F - Fox (6)

Rabies-positive animals in Michigan 1978–2000. (Michigan Department of Natural Resources. Redrawn by Jeff Dixon)

state of Michigan, usually acquired from dog bites. An extensive campaign to vaccinate dogs in Michigan against rabies was carried out in the mid 1950s. These programs dramatically decreased the number of rabies cases in domestic dogs.

The last case of human rabies in Michigan was reported in Hillsdale County in 1983 (CDC, 1983a). A 5-year-old female developed right arm pain and fever after a fall in February 7, 1883. An acute sprain of the right arm was diagnosed. She developed weakness, decreased appetite, sore throat, left heel pain, and right arm weakness in the next four days. She was hospitalized for further tests. She was alert and tenderness was noted at her right wrist, elbow, shoulder, and left heel. The white cell count in the blood was 12,800 (slightly elevated). She became progressively irritable with fever in the next 48 hours. The left arm weakness progressed and she also complained of difficulty in swallowing saliva and water. On February 13 she was more lethargic and her blood pressure was high. She was transferred to another hospital. CSF and a computed tomogram (CAT scan) of the brain were normal. The electroencephalogram (EEG) showed diffuse abnormality suggestive of encephalitis. She became less responsive and because of breathing difficulties she was connected to a respirator. High doses of steroids were given with a possible diagnosis of postinfectious encephalopathy (brain swelling that can occur after an infection, possibly resulting from a strong allergic reaction by the body). By February 17, she was comatose.

On February 23, the family remembered a possible bat bite in late August 1982. The blood samples and the CSF taken later in the course of the disease showed a rise in the rabies antibody titer and the diagnosis of rabies was confirmed. On March 9, 32 days after the onset of symptoms, the patient had a cardiac arrest and died. The rabies virus was identified in the brain at autopsy. Of the 254 persons at the two hospitals who had contact with potentially infectious secretions from the patient, 54 received postexposure prophylaxis.

Prior to this case, there had not been a case of human rabies in Michigan since 1948. Today, bats and skunks are the major carriers of rabies in Michigan, sometimes transmitting the virus to other species. Any rabid animal, regardless of its source of infection, can transmit rabies to humans. Dogs and cats are still frequently tested for rabies following bite incidents involving humans but they rarely test positive.

Bats are the animals most frequently testing positive for rabies in Michigan. The prevalence of rabies in Michigan's bat population is probably less than 1 percent; however, 4–6 percent of bats submitted for testing following a potential human or unvaccinated pet exposure test positive for rabies. This may be because rabid bats do not behave as their normal counterparts and might lose their way. More animals are submitted for testing in the spring. Potential rabies exposures and laboratory submissions are at their lowest levels in the winter. Geographically, bat rabies is generally widespread across the lower peninsula of Michigan, although cases do occur in the upper peninsula. Although terrestrial rabies in wild animals is mainly restricted to the southeastern region of the state, the identified cases of rabies are widespread across the state. The variety of animal species connected with rabies in Michigan is also interesting to note.

OTHER MODES OF TRANSMISISION

Rabies virus is transmitted when the virus is introduced into bite wounds or open cuts in skin or onto the mucous membranes. The likelihood of rabies infection varies with the nature and extent of exposure. Any penetration of the skin by the teeth of an animal constitutes a bite exposure. All bites, regardless of location, represent a potential risk of rabies transmission. Bites by some animals, such as bats, can inflict minor injury and thus be unnoticed. Non-bite exposures from terrestrial animals rarely cause rabies. However, occasional reports of transmission by non-bite exposure suggest that such exposures constitute sufficient reason to consider postexposure prophylaxis. The non-bite exposures of highest risk appear to be among persons exposed to large amounts of aerosolized rabies virus and surgical recipients of corneas transplanted from patients who died of rabies. Two cases of rabies have been attributed to probable aerosol exposures in laboratories, and a few cases of rabies have been attributed to possible airborne exposures in caves containing millions of free-tailed bats (*Tadarida brasiliensis*) in the southwest United States.

The contamination of open wounds, abrasions, mucous membranes, or scratches with saliva or other potentially infectious material (such as neural tissue) from a rabid animal also constitutes a non-bite exposure. Other contact by itself, such as petting a rabid animal and contact with blood, urine, or feces (e.g., guano) of a rabid animal, does not constitute an exposure and is not an indication for prophylaxis. Rabies virus is not present in these body fluids or secretions. Handling and skinning of the infected carcasses or even eating the infected meat has rarely resulted in transmission of rabies. Because the rabies virus is inactivated by desiccation and ultraviolet irradiation, in general, if the material containing the virus is dry, the virus can be considered noninfectious.

Aerosols in a Laboratory

Inhalation is another potential mode of transmission. It is implicated in the rabies transmission in caves. Although rare, caves harboring millions of bats have the potential for aerosolized rabies virus in the atmosphere. Laboratory transmission has also occurred by inhaling the aerosolized virus. In 1977, one of the researchers in a New York research laboratory was exposed to the aerosol of rabies virus while working with live rabies virus strains (Tillotson et al., 1977). He developed a prodrome of malaise, headache, and fever and then developed delirium. He had speech difficulties and was hyperreflexic. After admission to the hospital, he slipped into a coma. High viral titers were noted in the blood. After four months of hospitalization, he gradually improved and survived the disease. He was ambulatory, but was spastic and still has residual speech deficits. This is one of the six cases of rabies survived so far. He was given rabies vaccine derived from duck embryo cell lines as a part of the employment requirements. This might have played a part in the recovery of the patient.

Organ and Tissue Transplantation

Transplantation of the tissue is another mode of rabies transmission. The cornea has a rich nerve supply and rabies virus travels to the cornea from the brain via these nerve fibers. In fact, one of the diagnostic tests for rabies relies on this feature of the disease. Corneal impressions can be taken on a glass slide and then tested for the presence of rabies virus. Human-to-human transmission has occurred among eight recipients of transplanted corneas. Investigations revealed each of the corneal donors had died of an illness compatible with or proven to be rabies. The disease was not suspected in the diseased individuals before the corneas were harvested. The eight cases of rabies occurred in five countries: Thailand (two cases), India (two cases), Iran (two cases), the United States (one case), and France (one case). Since then, stringent guidelines for acceptance of donor corneas have been implemented to reduce this risk. The last of such cases was reported in 1994. Organ transplantation can also give rise to rabies. A case in Germany in 2004 resulted in the transmission of rabies to three of six organ transplant recipients. The original donor died suddenly because of an undetermined illness preceded by neuropsychiatric symptoms. The two kidney recipients and one pancreas transplant recipient developed rabies and died. A postmortem examination of the donor confirmed rabies as the cause of death.

Rabies Infections in Organ Donor and Transplant Recipients—Alabama, Arkansas, Oklahoma, and Texas, 2004

For the first time in the United States, three recipients of different solid organ transplant from a single donor were infected with rabies in May 2004 (Srinivasan, 2005). The organ donor was a 20-year-old Arkansas man who visited two hospitals in Texas. He presented with a change in mental status and a low-grade fever. A CAT scan of the brain was done and the diagnosis was bleeding under one of the outer coverings of brain (subarachnoid hemorrhage). The bleeding progressed rapidly in 48 hours and the patient became comatose. The pressure inside the skull increased and the patient died of brain herniation. This complication can occur in subarachnoid hemorrhage and the usual culprit of such a bleeding is rupture of an aneurysm inside the brain. Cocaine was found in the patient's system and doctors thought that the bleeding in the brain occurred because of the drug usage.

All potential organ donors in the United States are screened and tested for several infectious agents, and all require a virology screen to prevent possible transmission of infections from donor to recipient. Organ procurement organizations are responsible for evaluating organ donor suitability, consistent with minimum procurement standards. Organ donor eligibility is determined through a series of questions posed to family and contacts, physical examination, and blood testing looking for evidence of organ dysfunction. Tests for selected infections transmitted through blood are also performed. The virology screen includes testing for HIV (human immunodeficiency virus, responsible for causing AIDS), hepatitis B, hepatitis C, cytomegalovirus, human T-lymphotropic virus, toxoplasmosis, and syphilis. Rabies is not routinely tested before organ transplantation primarily because it is such a rare disease in the United States.

Donor eligibility screening and testing did not reveal any contraindications to transplantation in this patient. His family agreed to organ donation. The donor did not receive any blood products before death. Lungs, kidneys, and liver were recovered from the patient. The liver and the two kidneys were transplanted into three recipients on May 4 at a transplant center in Texas. The lungs were transported to an Alabama hospital where they were transplanted to another patient. This patient in Alabama died of intraoperative complications.

The three transplant recipients (the one liver and two kidney recipients) developed features of severe encephalitis of unknown etiology after the transplantation and subsequently died. Specimens were sent to the CDC for diagnostic evaluation. The following details the clinical course of the transplant recipients (CDC, 2004).

Liver Recipient

The liver was transplanted to a man with end-stage liver disease in Texas. He was discharged 5 days later after recovering from the surgery. Twenty-one days later he was re-admitted with general symptoms such as anorexia, tremors, and lethargy. During the next 24 hours, his mental status deteriorated rapidly and he became obtunded. He was admitted to the intensive care unit and connected to a respirator. Testing of the CSF revealed slightly increased white cell count and protein. His condition continued to deteriorate and was suggestive of rapidly progressive encephalitis. The patient subsequently died 56 days later. Specimens were sent to the CDC for evaluation of this unusual event following organ transplantation.

Female Kidney Recipient

The two kidneys were transplanted in two different individuals. The first kidney recipient was a woman with end-stage kidney failure caused by hypertension and diabetes. She also improved after the surgery and was discharged home on day 7. Twenty-five days after transplant, she complained of right flank pain. She underwent an appendectomy for this pain. Two days after this procedure, she developed diffuse twitching of muscles. She became lethargic and less responsive. A CAT scan and a magnetic resonance imaging of the brain did not reveal any abnormality. During the next 24–48 hours, the patient's condition worsened. She developed seizures, low blood pressure, and respiratory failure. She was intubated and connected to a respirator. Her condition did not improve at all and she developed swelling of the brain. The patient died after 2 weeks.

Male Kidney Recipient

The second kidney recipient was a man with end-stage kidney failure. He developed blockage of the artery of the transplanted kidney. This resulted in the infarction (death) of the lower pole of the transplanted kidney. This is not a life-threatening complication. The patient was discharged home 12 days after the surgery. He developed twitching of the muscles and change in mental status. He was re-admitted to the hospital. Brain scans were normal on admission. His condition deteriorated rapidly after admission. A study of the CSF showed mild elevations of the white cell count and protein in the fluid. He developed respiratory failure and was intubated and connected to a respirator. His condition did not improve. He developed progressive swelling of the brain and died after 10 days.

Laboratory Investigation

Samples were sent to the CDC from all the three patients. A histopathological examination of the brain showed evidence of inflammation (encephalitis). Characteristic viral inclusion bodies were seen under the microscope, suggesting

Negri bodies, which is diagnostic of rabies. Rabies was also confirmed in the brain by direct fluorescent antibody tests. Suckling mice inoculated intracranially and intraperitoneally with brain tissue from one kidney recipient died 7–9 days after the injection. The brain of the mice showed rabies virus. Further study of the virus showed similarity with rabies virus present in bats.

Fourth case of rabies

A liver transplant was done in a fourth patient the day after these transplants at the same hospital. A surgeon was trying to connect the transplanted liver from another donor to the recipient. The connecting artery was tiny and the surgeon used banked iliac artery. Unknown to the surgeon and others involved in the procedure, that artery came from the original donor. It was not known at that time that the donor had rabies and the other three recipients became infected through the transplanted organs. The fourth patient remained in the hospital with complications related to end-stage liver disease and died a few weeks later. Rabies was later diagnosed, but the patient did not show any symptoms of rabies because the patient was too sick from other complications.

Rabies virus antibodies were demonstrated in the blood from the original donor. It was not known how the donor contracted rabies. Subsequently it was found that he lived in an apartment complex in Texarkana where bats were often seen. Bat sightings were reported in the nearby areas as well. He had told others that he had been bitten by bats in the past.

Extremely Low Risk of Disease Transmission by Transplants

This report was the first documented cases of rabies virus transmission among solid organ transplant recipients. Rabies infection probably occurred through the neural tissue contained in these organs because rabies is not spread through blood contamination. This was a rare and unexpected event. The outbreak was only detected because of the astute observations of the pathologist and the officials involved. Several screening modalities practiced before organ donation significantly reduce and eliminate the chances of infection in most cases. Some risk is always present, but the object is to minimize the risk of infectious disease transmission to the lowest reasonably achievable level, without unduly decreasing the availability of this life-saving resource. The benefits from transplanted organs outweigh the minute risk for transmission of infectious diseases from screened donors.

Apart from corneal transplants, bite and non-bite exposures inflicted by infected humans with rabies manifestation could theoretically transmit rabies.

This could hypothetically happen in the furious stage of rabies when patients are agitated. Serious bites could be inflicted upon caregivers. Laboratory-diagnosed cases of rabies occurring under such situations have not been documented. Two nonlaboratory-confirmed cases of human-to-human rabies transmission have been described from Ethiopia. The route of exposure in both cases was direct salivary contact from another human (a bite and a kiss). Routine delivery of health care to a patient with rabies is not an indication for postexposure prophylaxis unless exposure of mucous membranes or non-intact skin to potentially infectious body fluids has occurred. Tissues or organs should never be transplanted from a patient who died of an undiagnosed neurological illness.

3

How Is Rabies Diagnosed?

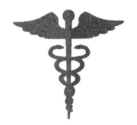

TWELVE-YEAR-OLD WITH RABIES

This is the story of an unnamed girl from one of the developing countries in Asia or Africa where rabies is widely prevalent. The 12-year-old girl and her family had a pet dog. The dog was not vaccinated and it roamed outside in its free time, becoming exposed to various other wildlife and stray dogs in the street. One day the girl was not feeling well and complained of muscle aches and pains. She also had numbness in one hand. Her parents took her to the local doctor and she was prescribed medications for a flu-like illness.

Her condition deteriorated during the next few days. She complained of difficulty in swallowing food. The family thought she was anxious about her upcoming examinations. She made a gasping noise and choked if a draft of air from a fan touched her. She was unable to swallow anything at all. The girl was taken to the emergency room where the physician took a brief history. Her difficulty in swallowing and inability to tolerate air from a fan made him suspect rabies. Upon further questioning, the family reported that while playing with her, the dog scratched her fingers few weeks ago.

The physician examined her and tried to fan her with a sheet of paper. The girl developed painful spasms of the neck muscles and choked. The same scenario was repeated when someone brought her a glass of water. This patient

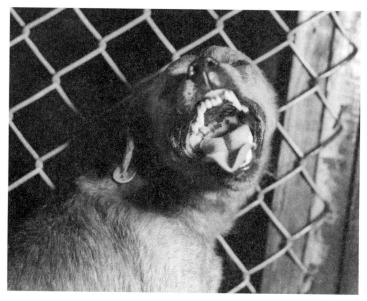

Dog suspected to have rabies. (CDC)

had two classical signs of rabies—aerophobia and hydrophobia. The next step to confirm a diagnosis of rabies would be to order further tests on the blood, cerebrospinal fluid, and the skin if facilities to do so are available.

Like any other disease, the diagnosis of rabies is dependent upon various tests. The presentation of the patient makes the physician suspect the possibility of rabies. Rabies is a neurotropic virus. After inoculation into the skin, it gains access to the sensory nerve fibers and travels unrelentingly to the spinal cord and eventually the brain.

CLINICAL FEATURES AND INCUBATION PERIOD

There is usually an *incubation period* before the disease manifests in humans. This is the time taken by the virus, after it is deposited in the subcutaneous tissue or the muscles by an animal bite, to multiply and travel to the brain. This time can vary, but usually human rabies manifests itself 20–90 days after exposure. Occasionally the disease develops after an interval of a few days. The reason for the wide variability in the incubation period is unknown. The reason for the documented longer incubation period in endemic countries may be a second exposure that may not be recollected by the patient or family because of the abundance of potential carriers such as stray animals. In general, severe multiple bites and bites in the face area have shorter incubation periods. This could be due to the high concentration of virus in the case of a severe bite. If a person is bitten on the face, the virus can possibly travel to the brain faster because of the close proximity. For example, a leg bite might take longer for the virus to travel through the peripheral nerves and the spinal cord to reach the brain.

The odds of a person developing rabies after a rabid animal bite are 50–80 percent after head bites, 15–40 percent after hand or arm bites, and 3–10 percent after leg bites. Several factors such as the density of the virus inoculum, the number of virus receptors, the degree of the innervation of the tissues, and the property of the rabies virus variant might affect whether a person is going to be infected after a bite.

First Symptoms of Rabies

The initial clinical features of rabies can be quite nonspecific and usually mimic a viral illness or flu-like illness. A high index of suspicion is needed in endemic areas not to miss this dreaded infection. The patient usually has fever, chills, fatigue, anorexia, headache, anxiety, and irritability. This might last for 10 days before the serious neurological features appear. Thirty to seventy percent of patients develop pain, paresthesia, or pruritus close to the site of the bite. These local manifestations may be more common in bat bites than with dog bites. Severe pain behind the eyes has been reported in cases of rabies occurring after corneal transplantation. Weakness can also occur in the bitten extremity. Again, this is more common with bat variants of the virus than with dog variants. The initial neurological symptoms rarely occur in a limb that was not bitten.

Classic (Furious) Rabies

In humans, 80 percent of the affected individuals exhibit the furious type of the disease. This type usually indicates a more aggressive form of the disease. The onset is triggered by the involvement of the brain with the rabies virus. Several mental changes such as confusion, agitation, and hallucinations can occur. These features can rarely lead to the diagnosis of a psychiatric illness in a patient with rabies. The patient also can have periods of hyperexcitability that are interspersed by relatively lucid periods. This hyperexcitability is an important feature of the disease. The hyperexcitable features can occur spontaneously or be precipitated by a variety of external stimuli such as auditory, visual, tactile, or olfactory stimuli.

The classic sign of rabies is *hydrophobia* (derived from Greek, meaning fear of water). About 50–80 percent of rabies patients develop hydrophobia and experience painful spasms of the throat muscles, making them unable to swallow anything. Attempts to swallow induce severe involuntary contractions of several muscles of the upper body, including the diaphragm (muscle separating the abdominal and chest cavities), sternomastoids (prominent muscle on the side of the neck), and other accessory muscles of respiration. These painful spasms last 5–15 seconds and can be followed by contractions of all of the neck muscles, resulting in the flexion or extension of the neck. These violent spasms can lead to vomiting, aspiration of food or saliva to the trachea, convulsions, or hypoxia (Jackson and Wunner, 2002, 223–225). Death can result from these spasms. Spasms can be terrifying, and later in the course of the disease the mere sight or even mention of water prompts such attacks. The patient avoids drinking water despite intense thirst. They become dehydrated and develop kidney failure. The reason for the hydrophobia is thought to be a selective infection of certain nerve cells controlling inspiration in the region of the nucleus ambiguous in the brainstem (Warrell, 1976). This could also indicate an exaggeration of the defensive reflexes to protect airways in normal individuals. This reflex acts as a conditioned response. Each episode of painful spasms upon trying to drink water reinforces the reflex in the victim's brain.

Another remarkable symptom in full-blown rabies is called "aerophobia" (Greek for fear of air). A gentle breeze, draft from a fan, or even the breath of an examiner can provoke such violent spasms. A fan test may be used at the bedside to confirm aerophobia. The resulting spasms can be painful and life threatening in the latter part of the disease. These spasms are basically due to the hyperexcitability of the nervous system that is affected by the infection by the virus.

These breathing patterns can worsen and the patient can have more frequent spasms, at shorter intervals, as the disease progresses. The amount of stimuli needed to precipitate such an attack also diminishes over time. The patient's breathing becomes more irregular, labored, and the level of consciousness also deteriorates.

The vocal cords can became weak and paralyzed, resulting in voice change and bark-like sounds. Other features like increased libido, priapism (painful erection), and spontaneous ejaculations have also been reported. Fever is also common. The autonomic nervous system, which controls the functions of various internal organs (such as heart and intestines) and is not under voluntary control, is also affected. Features such as excessive salivation, sweating, gooseflesh, and dilated pupils can be seen. The salivary volume can increase and drooling of saliva may occur because the patients cannot swallow their own saliva.

Because of the autonomic nervous system involvement, several cardiac complications are seen. These are important because the basic cardiac rhythm is altered and heart blocks can occur. Extra beats supervene and the heart will beat in a totally irregular manner. Blood pressure falls, the heart fails, and cardiac arrest can occur. Cardiac irregularity may be the reason for sudden death in rabies.

Temperature regulation of the body can be disturbed because of the involvement of the respective controlling areas in the brain. Both hyperthermia (high body temperature) and hypothermia (low body temperature) can be seen. Bleeding from the gastrointestinal tract, in the form of vomiting of blood, can occur and may even be terminal. Endocrine control can also be affected, resulting in the disturbance of the fluid electrolyte balance of the body, altering the constitution of the body chemicals.

Several cranial nerves can be paralyzed because of the infection. Cranial nerves controlling several bodily functions in the head and neck area can be affected. Paralysis of eye movements can ensue. The face can become asymmetric because of facial nerve paralysis. Tongue weakness can also occur in association with weakness of muscles of the pharynx, contributing to the dysphagia.

Ultimately, the patient becomes more obtunded and delirious. Gradual coma can intervene. Severe paralysis of muscles of the whole body also ensues. Multiple organs of the body, such as the heart, lungs, and kidneys, can fail.

Paralytic (Dumb) Rabies

Twenty percent of rabies patients present with the paralytic (dumb) form of the disease. The exact reason for the presentation is unknown. With this type, paralysis of the various muscles of the body develop relatively early in the course of the illness. This is not to be confused with the severe paralysis that can result in the later part of furious rabies. Weakness is prominent and it is usually confused with various other neurological illnesses causing weakness. This form of rabies is characterized by quieter clinical features as opposed to the furious variety. The laryngeal muscles can also be paralyzed, making the patent unable to talk. The predominance of the weakness masks the other terrifying features of furious rabies. The incubation period is similar and the weakness often starts in the extremity bitten by a rabid animal. It gradually spreads to the other extremities. The touch sensation is preserved.

The most common disease with which rabies is confused in the endemic areas is Guillain–Barré syndrome. This is an immunological reaction to a viral illness in which patients usually have weakness of the extremities and are unable to walk. The sensorium of the patient remains intact. Patients can die because of the involvement of respiratory muscles in Guillain–Barré syndrome.

This is not an infective condition and many patients recover with treatment. Sphincter involvement resulting in the loss of bladder control can occur in paralytic rabies, but not in Guillain–Barré syndrome.

Bat rabies is reported to have clinical features that differ from rabies spread by dog bites. Focal brainstem signs and myoclonus are more common in bat-associated rabies. Brainstem dysfunction results in weakness of muscles to the eyes, face, and neck, as well as disturbance of heart rhythm and breathing. Other signs described include weakness of one half of the body, sensory changes, ataxia, and abnormal movements.

Vampire bats have been associated with paralytic rabies outbreaks, most famously in the Caribbean island of Trinidad in the early 20th century. Seventy people were documented to have developed paralytic rabies from vampire bats on the island between 1929 and 1937. This disease was confused with other paralytic illnesses such as poliomyelitis and botulism. Rabies virus from vampire bats usually causes the paralytic form of the disease, predominantly in cattle. Rarely, this type of virus can also cause classic furious rabies, as exemplified by the rabies outbreak in Peru in the 1990s. This outbreak was characterized by several cases of human furious rabies from bat bites.

Da Rosa and colleagues reported two bat-transmitted outbreaks in remote rural areas of northern Brazil. Twenty-one persons died because of paralytic rabies in the two municipalities (da Rosa, 2006). Ten rabies virus strains were isolated from human specimens and two other cases were diagnosed by histopathological examination. Isolates were antigenically characterized as coming from the vampire bat *Desmodus rotundus*. Age of the patients ranged from 2 to 58 years. All patients reported receiving vampire bat bites several weeks or months before manifesting encephalitic symptoms. All patients exhibited a similar disease pattern, characterized by acute ascendant paralytic encephalitis.

The exact cause of these two types (furious and dumb varieties) with widely varying manifestations of a single disease is not known. Several theories are provided to explain this aberrancy. An earlier rise of antibody (proteins produced by the body to defend various infections) is seen in patients with classic rabies than in paralytic rabies. Patients with paralytic rabies could have defects in the immunological defenses of the body. This may mean a lack of lymphocytic response to the infection to fight it off. Lower levels of infection-fighting chemicals such as cytokines are also found in the paralytic variety. Alternatively, a focused attack of the rabies virus on the nerve roots supplying various muscles can result in paralytic rabies. The significance of these findings is speculative, and more research is needed to pinpoint the reason for this differing pathological manifestation of a disease caused by the same virus.

CLINICAL TESTS

After a thorough history and examination, doctors usually order various laboratory tests to confirm or refute the diagnosis of rabies. Some of the tests are relatively specific for rabies and some are rather nonspecific.

Usual Blood Tests

The usual blood tests such as a complete blood count and a metabolic panel can be normal in rabies because it is a viral infection, which usually does not cause any abrupt changes as might be seen in a bacterial infection. However, subtle changes such as an increase in the total white cell count with a predominance of lymphocytes may be observed. This is a very nonspecific finding and is probably not helpful in the diagnosis in most cases.

Specific Blood Tests

After the rabies virus has infected the nervous system, the human body mounts an immunological attack on the virus. The different cells in the body recognize the foreign antigen (virus) and mount an attack using different chemicals released from different parts of the immunological system. This reaction is useless for the most part because the rabies virus is strongly entrenched in the body cells, away from the blood stream, so these chemicals cannot penetrate the cells and damage the virus. However, this reaction is useful in identifying the presence of the virus. These serum "neutralizing antibodies" appear during the second week of the illness, but unfortunately the patient usually dies before a detectable level of the antibody is found in the blood samples. This severely limits its utility as a confirmatory test of rabies.

Cerebrospinal Fluid Studies

Cerebrospinal fluid (CSF) is present in the inside of the cranial cavity and the spinal column between the two membranes covering the brain and the spinal cord, known as the pia mater and the arachnoid membrane. This fluid is tested by doing a lumbar spinal puncture (lumbar tap). This test is a classical test to diagnose meningitis, an inflammation of the coverings of the brain. In bacterial meningitis, telltale evidence of a bacterial infection is found. White cells and protein in the fluid are high and glucose is low. The causative bacteria will grow in culturing the fluid. In contrast, viral illnesses will not produce any characteristic abnormalities in CSF. In rabies, like any viral illness, CSF findings can be nonspecific. Usually CSF contains only a small number of white cells. A mild increase in the number of white cells can be seen in rabies.

But this is only seen in 60 percent of the patients in the first week and 87 percent after the first week. Moreover, this test is also nonspecific and can be seen in a wide variety of viral illnesses. The protein in CSF may also be mildly elevated, and the glucose content is normal. The usefulness of these tests is not in confirming rabies, but in ruling out other potential illnesses such as bacterial meningitis. Rabies virus antibodies can also be tested in CSF. Unfortunately rabies virus antibodies develop later in CSF than in serum; the titers are low and difficult to measure.

Direct Detection of the Virus

In the above-mentioned techniques, the search is for surrogate markers of a viral infection. The ultimate diagnosis depends on finding the actual virus in the person or the tissue. The rabies virus is formed of RNA, and there are several techniques to detect the presence of RNA in various tissues. The most common specimens used for these tests are saliva, skin, cornea, CSF, and brain tissue. Ante-mortem identification of the rabies virus clinches the diagnosis and offers a glimmer of hope to start attempting a cure for the disease. One of the most common techniques used for this purpose is a biopsy of the skin of the back of the neck, known as nuchal biopsy. Full thickness punch biopsies are obtained from the hairy area of the nape of the neck. Care is taken to include hair follicles because rabies virus does show a predilection to affect the neurons beside hair follicles.

Different techniques can be used to pinpoint the presence of the rabies virus. One of the techniques is known as the direct fluorescent antibody (DFA) technique in the frozen samples of the skin biopsy. This is the most reliable test to confirm the diagnosis of rabies. To perform this test, at first laboratory animals are sensitized with the rabies virus. These animals produce antibody in their blood against rabies. Antibodies are isolated from the animals' blood and joined chemically in the laboratory with a fluorescent dye. This antibody-dye complex will glow brightly under ultraviolet light, and the complex is known as the fluorescent antibody (Parker and Parker, 2002, 20). The fluorescent antibodies are mixed with the sample of the tissue in question. The fluorescent antibody binds with the rabies virus in the tissue and shows up as a fluorescent glow under the microscope. This test can be used in skin biopsy specimens or sections of the brain. A fluorescent antibody test can be used to diagnose rabies in both humans and animals.

Negri Bodies

In the past, scientists demonstrated Negri bodies to diagnose rabies. Adelchi Negri, an Italian physician, pathologist, and microbiologist, originally discovered Negri bodies in 1903. Negri consistently found these structures in the brain of diseased animals, but mistakenly thought that they represented a parasite that caused rabies. The fact that rabies is caused by a virus was discovered by Alfonso Di Vesta in Naples, and Paul Remlinger at Riffat Bey in Constantinople a few months later. Negri bodies are clumps of the RNA virus in the nerve cells where they multiply. Negri bodies can be detected in hematoxylin-eosin stained samples of the brain tissue under the microscope as a pink object. They average in size from 1–20 μm and are seen as round, oval, or spindle-shaped objects inside the neurons (Jackson and Wunner, 2002, 286–287). They are most characteristically seen in the Ammon's horn region of the hippocampus. The demonstration is cumbersome and includes a postmortem examination of the brain; therefore, to make a diagnosis the animal has to be sacrificed. Less cumbersome and easier antemortem diagnostic tests are popular because of these reasons. Another important caveat is that Negri bodies can be absent in 20 percent of patients, therefore absence of Negri bodies does not necessarily rule out rabies.

Corneal Imprint

A corneal imprint is made on a glass slide by pressing the slide gently on the cornea of the patient. The material on the slide can then be tested for the presence of the rabies virus. The cornea may be a difficult area to sample, especially in a comatose patient. One complication of the procedure is permanent damage to the cornea. Because of this, only a trained ophthalmologist in consultation with the testing laboratory should do the procedure. The sample is collected by rubbing a slide on each cornea. These slides can tested with the DFA technique or reverse transcriptase polymerase chain reaction (RT-PCR) to detect the presence of the virus.

Detection of Rabies Virus RNA

Polymerase chain reaction (PCR) is another test used to identify rabies virus in specimens. PCR is a technique by which the DNA samples in the tissue are amplified using special enzymes and techniques to identify a viral DNA. A subtle variation of this test, known as RT-PCR, is used to detect RNA viruses (Jackson, 2000). In this test, rabies virus RNA is amplified into several copies that can be identified. Although this test is highly sensitive, currently the World Health Organization (WHO) does not recommend it to confirm the diagnosis of rabies after death. This may be used to diagnose the disease antemortem; however, significant false-positive or false-negative tests can occur. Therefore this test should only be used in conjunction with other tests for the highest diagnostic accuracy. It is also recommended that in attempts to diagnose rabies, both saliva and skin specimens be obtained for testing because rabies virus may be positive only in a certain percentage of either specimen.

Virus Isolation

One of the most common confirmatory tests used is the cultivation of the virus by inoculation of the material into a test laboratory animal or cell line. The mouse inoculation test is reliable for this purpose. A small piece of the brain is homogenized by a mortar and pestle in a buffered saline diluent containing protein stabilizer and antibiotics. Five laboratory mice are injected intracerebrally with the specimen and observed for the next 30 days. Mice that develop signs of rabies are sacrificed and their brains are tested for the presence of rabies virus by DFA.

Virus isolation also can be done using a cell culture line. Cell cultures are thin layers of live cells in the laboratory that can be infected with a variety of infective agents. A murine neuroblastoma cell line is used to detect the presence of rabies virus. Tissue culture flasks or plates are seeded with the host cells and the cells are incubated for several days. Cells are then examined for evidence of rabies virus infection using DFA.

Other Tests

The usual imaging studies such as X-rays and computed scans (CT or CAT scans) of the brain are normal in rabies. The more advanced MRI (magnetic resonance imaging) studies have been obtained in a few cases, mostly done to investigate the cause of unknown encephalitis that turned out to be rabies discovered after the patient's death. These MRI scans showed both normal findings and increased T-2 weighted images in the medulla and pons. Lighting up of the spinal nerve roots with contrast agents are reported in one case of paralytic rabies. These tests are nonspecific and do not help in the diagnosis of rabies. The cost and availability are also concerns, especially in developing countries. Similarly, brain wave mapping or EEG (electroencephalogram) may also be normal or show nonspecific abnormalities such as slow wave activity.

Antemortem Diagnosis in Humans

Diagnosis of rabies should be considered in patients presenting with encephalopathy of undetermined origin in the right setting. As detailed earlier, antemortem diagnosis of rabies in humans is one of the most difficult diagnoses to make. A battery of tests is used. In case of suspicion, an experienced laboratory should be contacted. Health care personnel should consult with the state health department or the rabies laboratory of the Centers for Disease Control and Prevention (CDC) in Atlanta, Georgia. The samples should he collected and frozen to a temperature of -20°C or below. Samples should be shipped by overnight courier in dry ice, and the laboratory should be informed of the exact details of shipping so samples can be retrieved and processed in a timely manner.

Saliva can be used to detect the presence of the rabies virus RNA by RT-PCR. Saliva is collected in a sealed container without preservatives. Saliva contains a large number of virus particles. The skin biopsy specimens usually taken from the nape of the neck should be placed on a sterile piece of gauze and moistened with saline or sterile water in a container. Neck skin biopsy specimens are tested for virus RNA by RT-PCR or immunofluorescent staining. A small amount (0.5 mL) of serum or CSF is needed for testing for antibodies. The presence of antibody in a nonimmunized individual is diagnostic of the disease. Corneal imprint is another method used to diagnose rabies antemortem. Brain biopsy is rarely used to diagnose rabies antemortem. Rabies should be tested in samples being tested for other infections in case of undiagnosed encephalitis. RT-PCR and immunofluorescent staining are the methods of choice in this regard. To make a diagnosis of rabies postmortem in humans, the brain material obtained during an autopsy can be submitted for the DFA test, which will give immediate results. The other alternative is to test the formalin-fixed brain tissue for the presence of Negri bodies under the microscope.

Rabies Diagnosis in Wild and Domestic Animals

Rabies diagnosis in animals helps to streamline resources. Evidence of rabies infection in an animal prompts timely administration of postexposure prophylaxis with rabies vaccine in individuals bitten or exposed to the virus. This also helps in the prompt management of exposed domestic animals. Animals that were previously inoculated with the virus can be given booster doses of the vaccine. Previously unvaccinated animals could be quarantined or euthanized. Reliable negative results from the diagnostic tests will avert unnecessary and costly postexposure prophylaxis to the exposed individuals or animals.

The most common diagnostic test used in the diagnosis of rabies in animals is the DFA test. This test is done postmortem on the animal's brain, after the rabid animal is dead or sacrificed. The virus first travels to the infected animal, populating its brain, and subsequently travels down along the nerves to the salivary gland and the saliva. Because of this, testing the brain of a rabid animal will give a definite clue to the diagnosis.

Not all animals that bite or scratch need to be killed in countries with excellent rabies prevention programs. Biting incidents involving healthy dogs, cats, or ferrets are common, but no case of rabies from such cases has been reported in North America. The public health recommendation is to quarantine and observe such animals for 10 days. The animal does not need to be killed and tested unless it shows signs and symptoms of rabies within this observation period. No prophylaxis is initiated for the person bitten. In rabies-endemic areas with poor rabies control programs, rabies vaccination is started along with the quarantine and stopped at the end of the observation period if the animal is healthy. This 10-day observation period is not suitable for animals already showing signs of rabies or wild or exotic species. In these situations the animals should be humanely euthanized and tested for the virus. Testing is also suggested in the following circumstances even if a bite or contact did not occur:

1. Bats captured in close indoor environments because a bat bite may go unrecognized and put the individuals living in the area at risk.
2. Domestic animal dying with probable signs of rabies.
3. Animals that are not usually infected with rabies such as bear, deer, and beaver that present with neurological symptoms of rabies.
4. Symptomatic rabid animals captured beyond the known geographical prevalence of that particular species.
5. Animals caught from the area where preventive measures such as oral vaccination programs are being carried out. This is done to assess the efficacy of such strategies.

OTHER DIFFERENTIAL DIAGNOSES OF RABIES

The diagnosis of rabies can be difficult, especially if a clear exposure history is lacking or forgotten by the patient. The early features might mimic psychiatric illnesses such as schizophrenia, psychosis, or mania. In endemic areas, especially in the developing world, first-time diagnosis of those psychiatric illnesses should be done with due diligence. Other viral encephalitis infections such as herpes simiae encephalomyelitis can also mimic rabies. This disease is transmitted by monkey bites. Hydrophobia is absent in other types of encephalitis. Vesicles might be present at the site of monkey bites in case of herpes simiae encephalitis.

Tetanus is caused by the neurotoxin of the bacterium *Clostridium tetani.* Tetanus can develop after an animal bite because of the contamination of a dirty wound by tetanus spores. It has a shorter incubation period. Unlike rabies, tetanus is characterized by continuous muscle rigidity. The central or axial muscles are involved, causing tonic posturing and stiffening of the body. Recurrent muscle spasms can occur, but sensorium is unaffected in tetanus and the patient remains lucid. Prognosis is generally better than rabies.

In patients who received postexposure prophylaxis with the older type of vaccine, vaccine complications can occur. One of the common reactions to the vaccine is called "postvaccinal encephalomyelitis." This is an immunological reaction to the neural tissue in the vaccine. Symptoms can resemble an encephalomyelitis, with changes in the sensorium, confusion and even weakness because of the involvement of spinal cord. Local symptoms at the site of the bite, alternating agitation and lucidity, and hydrophobia are absent in these cases. The presence of those signs favors the diagnosis of rabies rather than postvaccinal illness.

Paralytic rabies can also mimic Guillain–Barré syndrome. Local symptoms at the site of the animal bite, piloerection, early urinary bladder dysfunction, and fever are more common in paralytic rabies. CSF examination might give more clues regarding Guillain–Barré syndrome. Rabies can also mimic several other neurological illnesses such as poliomyelitis, stroke, brain tumors, and epilepsy. Confusion regarding the diagnosis can occur in developing countries where the prevalence of these neurological illnesses far outnumbers the cases of rabies. Diagnosis may be made only when the patient develop obvious signs of rabies such as hydrophobia or aerophobia. These are clinical tests that can be performed at the bedside to suspect rabies. In developing countries rabies may also be diagnosed as psychosis during the initial illness when the patient exhibits behavioral changes. Paralytic rabies may be mistaken for the depressed sullen stupor of psychosis, and the patient might end up in a psychiatric ward. All of those initial assumptions will expose several healthcare workers and other family members to potential rabies.

The definitive diagnosis of rabies is very important because of the serious nature of the disease. Several of the conditions described above could be treated with different modalities of treatments. In the case of rabies, there are no proven cures. Prompt measures taken immediately after exposure to a rabid animal in the form of a vaccine remain the best strategy to prevent this illness.

4

Prevention of Rabies

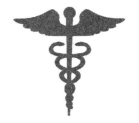

Chance favors only the prepared mind.

—Louis Pasteur

THE STORY OF LOUIS PASTEUR

Rabies is a deadly, uniformly fatal disease with few exceptions. The only silver lining is that prompt postexposure prophylaxis is extremely effective in preventing the disease, even after being bitten by a rabid animal. The protocol uses a combination of vaccine and immune globulin. The story of this proven method starts in the 1880s and we owe it to the ingenuity of the French scientist Louis Pasteur.

Louis Pasteur was one of the most brilliant minds in the history of science. Born into ordinary circumstances in rural France, he developed an interest in crystallography in Paris and made landmark discoveries about the different forms of tartaric acid crystals. He was a professor of chemistry, but his interests included fermentation and silk worms. He helped one of the factories in Paris to perfect the techniques of fermentation so that they were able to make alcohol instead of lactic acid. Next, the French government commissioned him to explore the cause of the devastating disease of silk worms that was destroying

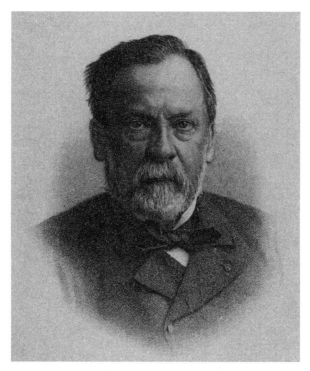

Louis Pasteur, who administered the first vaccine against rabies. (Library of Congress)

the French silk industry. Pasteur formulated a method to eliminate the diseased sick silk worms and grow healthy ones in the nursery. Later, Pasture performed research on anthrax bacterium and chicken cholera.

Serendipitous Finding of a Vaccine for Chicken Cholera

Serendipitously Pasteur and his team discovered that cultures of chicken cholera bacterium were not able to infect the chickens if they were stored for some time. But interestingly, if subsequent virulent cultures were administered to those chickens, nothing happened; all of the chickens survived. On the contrary, the birds that were given the virulent cultures for the first time died. This was an exciting idea: Injection of an attenuated (weak) strain of the bacteria could lead to the development of resistance to the infection. Pasteur applied this theory to anthrax and succeeded.

Pasteur Develops the First Rabies Vaccine

Pasteur turned his attention to rabies. Rabies was a dreaded disease in those times. Rabies was associated with visions of raging victims, bound and howling, or asphyxiated between two mattresses. The treatment applied to the unfortunate victims was also brutal. This included cauterization of the wound with a red-hot poker. Pasteur and colleagues tried to transfer the disease using the saliva from infected dogs, but this was unreliable. So, with meticulous technique they figured out that the extracts of spinal cords of rabid animals could cause the disease if injected directly into the brain of the dogs. Pasteur thought of developing a vaccine to protect the brain before the rabies virus traveled to brain tissue from the peripheral nerves. He knew that the spinal cord of laboratory animals infected with rabies contained the infective agent. Spinal cords of rabid rabbits were dried in air to reduce the potency of the virus. A longer drying time decreased the potency of the specimen (Robbins, 2001, 95). This material was injected under the skin of the test animal every day in increasing potencies to impart immunity to that animal. Stronger and stronger doses of the extract were given for the next 12 days. At the end of the experiment the animals became resistant to rabies. They did not contract the disease even if bitten by rabid dogs. Even direct injection of the rabid material directly into their brains failed to cause the disease.

This discovery was amazing and widely publicized. It is worthwhile to note that Pasteur made his discovery entirely on intuition and thorough observation. He did not know that a virus caused rabies at that time. The infective agent of rabies remained elusive. The public wanted Pasture to test the cure for dogs in humans. Pasteur was terribly afraid and wanted several years more research to isolate the rabies agent before starting human experiments.

The First Recipient of Rabies Vaccine: Joseph Meister

New events unfolded in 1886. As public pressure increased to test the vaccine in humans, Pasteur was preparing to test the vaccine on himself. The Emperor of Brazil wrote to him asking if the vaccine could be given to humans. On July 6, 1885, 9-year-old Joseph Meister and his mother presented themselves before Pasteur. The boy was walking to school on the previous day, and a dog ran towards him in the field and knocked him down. The dog was rabid and the boy was bitten 14 times on the hands, body, and over the face. The dog was killed. Joseph was taken to his local doctor and he cauterized the wounds with carbolic acid, as was the practice. He told Joseph's family that the only person who could save his life was Louis Pasteur.

Joseph's mother pleaded with Pasteur to administer his vaccine to Joseph. Pasteur saw the boy's agony and he knew certain death was in store for the boy if he did not intervene. He had a detailed discussion with the family about the potential for things to go awry. He said the vaccine might even infect the boy with rabies. Joseph's mother was persistent. Pasteur was not a medical doctor; he was a chemist by trade. Louis Pasteur asked for the advice of two of his physician friends. The doctors thought the wound was cauterized 12 hours after the dog bite. They did not give the boy any chance at all. Moreover, the wound was showing signs of infection.

Louis Pasteur decided to administer the vaccine to Joseph Meister. The vaccine was prepared from the brain substance of a rabbit infected with rabies. A few drops of liquid containing fragments of the brain were injected into Joseph's right abdominal wall. Pasteur was not at all sure whether this would work for Joseph. Each morning he dreaded that Joseph might come down with rabies. But every morning Joseph was healthy and the injections continued. The wounds started to heal. Joseph received 13 injections of the vaccine in 11 days.

By mid-August of 1885, Joseph Meister was still healthy, and the wounds healed. There were no signs of rabies. Pasture wrote "Joseph is yet well and seems recovered from his wounds. It has been thirty-one days since he was bitten. *He is now quite safe. The vaccine is successful*" (Dolan, 1958, 203).

A few months later, Pasture treated another victim of a rabid dog attack. His name was Jean Baptiste Jupille. He was a shepherd and was attacked by a mad dog while trying to protect his friends. He presented to Pasteur 7 days after the attack. Pasteur was skeptical because of the delay. However, the boy survived with the help of rabies vaccine injections.

Worldwide Acclaim

Pasteur won worldwide acclaim for his accomplishments. Victims of dog and wolf bites from France, Russia, and the United States poured into his laboratory in Paris. The *New York Herald* raised money through public subscription to send four American children bitten in the "Newark dog scare" to Paris to be vaccinated. Pasteur became a hero and a legend. The Pasteur Institute was built in Paris with contributions from the public and the government to conduct research in various infectious diseases. Several Pasteur Institutes were opened worldwide with donations and help from philanthropists and leading scientists. By the time Pasteur died in 1895, about 20,000 people had received rabies vaccines all over the world (Geison, 1995, 218).

The First Vaccine Derived from Neural Tissue

The Pasteur rabies vaccine derived from neuronal tissue remained the cornerstone of rabies treatment for several decades. During the initial years, several methods of vaccine production were attempted, and they all used infected neuronal tissue. The rabies vaccine forms an integral part of the postexposure prophylaxis.

Vaccine Innovations

In the early 1900s Fermi and Semple introduced two innovations in the making of the vaccine. They inactivated the rabies-infected brain with phenol and used the same strength of the vaccine for all the injections (Jackson and Wunner, 2002, 372). Semple vaccine is produced from sheep brain. Very young sheep are injected intracerebrally with the rabies virus derived from the original Pasteur strain. The animals are euthanized 6–7 days later at the onset of clinical symptoms of rabies. The brains are removed, homogenized, and inactivated with phenol. The solution is filtered to remove large particles and filled in vials. The shelf life of the vials is only 6 months and they may not be effective afterwards. The dose is 2 mL for children and 5 mL for adults. Because of the volume of the injection, they are usually administered into the abdominal wall. The skin is pinched and the injection is given under the skin. This can be very painful because of the volume of the vaccine. The number of doses required varies from 7 to 15. The presence of myelin in the Semple vaccine can cause severe complications in the vaccine recipients. The myelin is the covering of the neuronal cells and usually develops after birth. Myelin is a foreign protein and can cause severe reactions in certain patients. The most important and dangerous complication is known as vaccine-induced encephalomyelitis, manifested by mental status changes and severe paralysis. These symptoms can occur in as many as 1 in 150 recipients of the vaccine in some instances. These symptoms can also mimic rabies, causing confusion in the diagnosis. The injection of sheep-brain-derived vaccine also puts the recipients at risk for the transmission of other slow viral diseases such as spongiform encephalopathy seen in sheep (Jackson and Wunner, 2002, 374).

Suckling Mouse Vaccine

To avoid the presence of myelin in the vaccine, newborn mice were used for vaccine production in the 1950s. Newborn mice lack myelin since myelin is deposited in the brain during the first few weeks of life. Suckling mouse vaccine lacks myelin and is still used in Latin America. These neuronal-cell-based vaccines are easier and cheaper to produce and are widely used in developing countries. Mice no more than a day old are inoculated in the brain with the virus and the brain tissue is harvested approximately 4 days later (Jackson and Wunner, 2002, 375). Although the rate of adverse reactions is less in the suckling mouse brain vaccine, significant morbidity is still noted with this vaccine.

Because of the high incidence of neurological complications, the World Health Organization (WHO) mandated in 2001 that modern cell culture vaccines replace all neural tissue-derived vaccines.

The first non-neuronal rabies vaccine was the duck embryo vaccine that was available in the United States in 1957. This vaccine was developed using duck embryo cell lines. Although this vaccine caused significantly fewer neurological complications, 21 serious neurological complications, including two deaths, were reported between 1958 and 1975.

Modern Cell Culture Vaccines

Cell cultures are layers of live cells, maintained in the laboratory and taken from various tissues of different animals or human beings. These cell lines are kept alive by supplying nutrients. This medium is ideal for culturing viruses because of their propensity to infect cells and use of the cellular machinery for replication. The first cell culture vaccine was the human diploid cell vaccine (HDCV) introduced in the United States in 1978. The virus is harvested from infected human diploid cells (the MRC-5 strain), concentrated by ultrafiltration, and inactivated by beta propiolactone. The vaccine should be used immediately after reconstitution otherwise potency may be lost. Instead of the usual 7–15 injections required for neural tissue-derived vaccine, cell culture vaccine needs only five injections after rabies exposure. Only three injections are needed for pre-exposure prophylaxis in high-risk individuals. This vaccine can also be injected into the topmost layer of the skin (dermis) as an intradermal injection. This decreases the quantity of the vaccine used. This vaccine elicits a satisfactory antibody response, with seroconversion often obtained after only one dose. With two doses 1 month apart, 100 percent of the recipients developed specific antibody against rabies. Side effects to the vaccine may include pain, redness, and swelling or itching at the injection site; headache, nausea, and abdominal pain are also possible. Frequent booster doses in high-risk individuals can also produce a severe allergic reaction therefore the policy of administering routine boosters was changed. The current policy is to test for the level of neutralizing antibody in the blood and give the vaccine if the levels are low. The cost of this cell culture vaccine may be prohibitive in developing countries.

In the 1980s a second cell culture vaccine was produced from primary chick fibroblast cell lines. Purified chick embryo cell rabies vaccine can be produced on a massive scale and has fewer adverse reactions than the neural vaccine. This vaccine is used worldwide.

A recent innovation in rabies vaccine production involves the use of continuous cell lines that can be multiplied and passed on serially for an unlimited number of times. This makes the production of the vaccine easier. The most reliable vaccine produced from a continuous cell line is purified Vero cell vaccine produced on Vero cells isolated from kidney epithelial cells extracted from African green monkeys. Large quantities of the vaccine can be produced at a lower costs than the human diploid cell vaccine. This is not licensed in North America, but is used in Europe. Another vaccine licensed in the United States is the RVA (rabies vaccine adsorbed), produced in the 1970s by the Michigan Department of Public Health by infecting fetal rhesus monkey kidney cells with rabies virus.

Rabies Vaccines for Animals

The estimated total annual expenditure for rabies prevention amounts to $300 million in the United States. Widespread vaccine for domestic dogs is the time-tested preventive measure for rabies. The United States has recently eradicated the canine rabies virus; however, this does not alleviate the need for continued vaccination. Domestic dogs in this country could potentially be infected by any number of wild animals that can carry rabies virus. Therefore it is very important to keep up with the vaccination of domestic animals. If the vaccination rates of the susceptible hosts are in the 70 percent range, there is a hope for control of this epidemic. This is still an unattainable goal in many parts of the world, especially in the developing world. Stray dogs are a pressing issue in several parts of the world because they maintain a cycle of canine rabies and also act as susceptible hosts for the virus to infect from the wild cycle through wild animal bites.

Local governments usually oversee effective programs to ensure vaccination of all dogs, cats, and ferrets and to remove strays and unwanted animals. As a result, laboratory-confirmed cases of rabies in dogs have decreased from 6,949 in 1947 to 117 in 2003 in the United States. Vaccination of cats should be required because there are more cases of rabies in cats (321 in 2003) than dogs. Animal shelters and animal control authorities should establish policies to ensure that adopted animals are vaccinated against rabies. Effective rabies vaccines are available for dogs, cats, ferrets, sheep, cattle, and horses. Vaccination of cats and dogs is crucial, because vaccinated pets are a protective barrier between the people who own and interact with them and rabid wild animals with which the pets might have contact. Even if the pet owners consider their pets as "indoor animals," they should still be vaccinated because of the potential for outside contacts with other animals or even contacts with bats. The curiosity of the animals increases their risks for such exposure. A licensed veterinarian must administer vaccinations. Primary and booster vaccinations should be obtained in accordance with recommendations from licensed veterinarians and in accordance with local animal control ordinances for prophylaxis. There is no postexposure treatment available for animals as there is for humans.

Peak rabies antibody titer is reached within 28 days after primary vaccination and the animal can be considered immunized. A booster vaccination should be administered 1 year later. There is no need to repeat the vaccinations. Pasteur originally used inactivated vaccines in animals. Just as in humans, neuronal cell-derived inactivated vaccines were used in dogs for several decades, but they caused several neuroparalytic complications and several animals perished because of complications of the vaccine rather than of rabies. Other mediums such as embryonated chicken eggs were used to produce the vaccine subsequently. Several passages through serial culture lines reduced the potency of the virus and the immunized dogs were safe. This vaccine occasionally caused rabies in cats, young pups, and cattle. Further passages in the cell culture until there was absolutely no evidence of infectivity mitigated this complication.

Vaccine Potency and Schedule

There are several killed, or inactivated, vaccines on the market. A variety of methods to inactivate/kill the virus and produce the vaccine are used, depending on the manufacturer. Various cell lines are used to grow the virus and several chemicals are used to inactivate the virus. The most common inactivating agent used today is beta propiolactone (BPL). Once inactivated, substances known as adjuants are added to the vaccine to increase the potency. Federal authorities ensure the safety and efficacy of these inactivated vaccines. The National Institutes of Health (NIH) came up with a test to measure the potency of the inactivated vaccine in 1974. This was necessary because of vaccine failure in early days, resulting in vaccinated animals contracting rabies. The NIH test is the gold standard for ensuring the potency of inactivated rabies vaccine in the United States. The inactivated vaccines should be administered to the animals at 3 months of age and repeated after 1 year. Depending on the vaccine, animal species, and local regulations, the animals must be vaccinated annually or triennially thereafter. The compendium released by the Centers for Disease Control and Prevention (CDC) in 2005 regarding animal rabies control also states that there are no laboratory or epidemiologic data to support the annual or biennial administration of 3-year vaccines following the initial series. Because a rapid anamnestic response is expected, an animal is considered currently vaccinated immediately after a booster vaccination (CDC, 2005). An anamnestic response consists of a more rapid production of antibodies in larger amounts that last for a longer time. This is mediated by specialized immune cells in the body that can "remember" the foreign antigen.

Live viruses can also be modified and adapted for different cell culture mediums such as hamster kidney tissue. There are several variations of this type of vaccine and they are used extensively in Europe and Asia for animal inoculation. Some of these vaccines are adapted for oral vaccination of animals. Oral vaccination is a promising technique to increase vaccination rates in animals, especially stray dogs, in several parts of the world. Vaccine baits are used to vaccinate them because the parenteral administration of a vaccine is either impossible or a costly endeavor. None of the modified live vaccines are licensed to use in the United States.

Rabies is a very rare event after vaccination in animals. If such a diagnosis is suspected, state and federal authorities should be informed and all attempts undertaken to obtain a correct diagnosis. The vaccine manufacturer also should be informed.

Oral Vaccines for Wildlife—Europe

Ambitious projects to vaccinate free ranging animals in the wild with rabies vaccine were first attempted in European countries in the 1980s. Modified virus strains were used in these intense field trials. The virus was inserted inside fat or fishmeal baits and wild animals such as foxes that ate the bait were immunized unknowingly. Rabies was eradicated in Europe during the early parts of the 20th century by widespread immunization of dogs and destruction of wild packs of dogs. Rabies sprang up again on the Russian/Polish border in the 1930s. World War II helped the disease spread by allowing packs of unvaccinated dogs to roam loose. Dogs and foxes contracted rabies from this 'reservoir' among wild animals in Russia. Dog rabies was controlled again in the late 1940s. The infection established itself in foxes in the wild, and started spreading as a major epizootic. Fox rabies has since spread west through Europe at a rate of 30 to 40 kilometers per year. Because of geographical continuity, it reached West Germany in 1950, Belgium in 1966, and western France in 1989. Food pellets packed with the vaccine can be airdropped in the wild (European Commission, 2002). The Belgians carried out two aerial vaccinations during the cold season (November and March) when the fox population density is at its lowest. Control of aerial distribution of the vaccine baits was intensified by use of GPS (Global Positioning System) and reducing the distance between flight lines to 500 meters. The baiting density was increased from 15 to 17 baits per km^2.

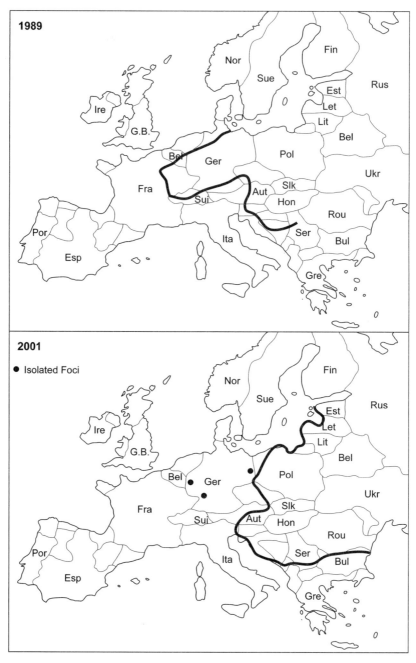

Western limits of wild life rabies in Europe in 1989 and 2001. (*Rabies Bulletin Europe*
1989–2001. Redrawn by Jeff Dixon)

Such drastic control measures had a dramatic impact on the incidence of rabies in Germany as well. The number of wild animals with rabies in Germany plummeted from 10,487 in 1983 to 83 cases in 1997. These attempts have decisively pushed back the western limits of the rabies endemic much further to the east, and stopped the spread of the disease in the wild except for a few pockets of isolated cases.

In Europe, several methods of bait distribution have been adopted. Manual distribution is carried out in certain areas. For large-scale distribution, either helicopters or fixed wing aircrafts have been used. Another advance in wild animal vaccination is the development of the recombinant rabies vaccine. In this method, the attenuated rabies virus vaccine strain is piggybacked onto another virus known as a vector. The virus usually used in this method is the Copenhagen strain of the vaccinia virus. A portion of the gene of the rabies virus was inserted into the genomic material of this virus, and the recombinant virus was produced. This virus was found to be very effective in protecting wild animals from rabies in field tests. There was some concern regarding its safety, but to date no adverse effects have been reported. In 1995, the United States Department of Agriculture (USDA) licensed an oral rabies vaccine for restricted use in oral immunization of raccoons in the United States.

PRE-EXPOSURE PROPHYLAXIS IN HUMANS

Individuals Offered Pre-Exposure Prophylaxis

Pre-exposure prophylaxis is the preventative administration of rabies vaccine to people or populations at risk of contracting rabies before any kind of exposure. Pre-exposure vaccination for rabies should be offered to people at high risk for exposure, such as those working in rabies diagnostic or research laboratories, veterinarians, animal handlers (including bat handlers), animal rehabilitators and wildlife officers, as well as other people (especially children) living in or traveling to high-risk areas. Children under 15 years represent approximately 50 percent of human exposures in canine rabies-infected areas. Vaccines produced in cell culture or from embryonated eggs should be used for pre-exposure vaccination of humans. It is important to remember that pre-exposure treatment of rabies using a vaccine does not preclude more definite treatment in case of an exposure. However, pre-exposure prophylaxis given properly will alleviate the need for other interventions such as administration of the immune globulins after an exposure. Those persons might also require a fewer number of rabies vaccine injections after an exposure.

The two types of vaccines available in the United States for pre-exposure prophylaxis are human diploid cell vaccine (HDCV) and purified chick embryo cell vaccine (PCEC). The trade name for human diploid cell vaccine (HDCV) is Imovax®, produced by Sanofi Pasteur SA which is a sterile, stable, freeze-dried suspension of rabies virus prepared from strain PM-1503-3M obtained from the Wistar Institute, Philadelphia, Pennsylvania. This cell culture rabies vaccine contains no preservatives or stabilizers. Purified chick embryo cell vaccine (PCEC) is marketed as RabAvert® and is produced by Chiron Behring GmbH and company. This is a sterile freeze-dried vaccine obtained by growing the fixed-virus strain Flury low egg passage (LEP) in primary cultures of chicken fibroblasts.

Primary vaccination is carried out by administering three 1.0-mL injections of HDCV or PCEC vaccine intramuscularly. One injection per day is given on days 0, 7, and 21 or 28. A few days' variation is acceptable. The vaccine is administered into the upper arm (deltoid region) of adults and into the antero-lateral (the side) thigh region of young children. The vaccine should never be administered into the gluteal region because absorption is unpredictable. Vaccine preparations for intradermal administration are no longer available in the United States.

Rabies research laboratory workers and rabies biologics production workers are considered high risk. The virus is present in their work environment at a high concentration and specific exposures may go unnoticed (CDC, 2007a). Bite, non-bite, or aerosol exposures are all possibilities. They are given the primary course of three injections of the vaccine and offered serological testing every 6 months. If the serological levels of rabies antibody titers are found to be low, they should be offered booster doses. The first category of people who are advised routine pre-exposure prophylaxis includes rabies diagnostic laboratory workers, spelunkers, veterinarians and staff, as well as animal-control and wildlife workers in rabies-enzootic areas. The second category includes all persons who frequently handle bats and are at risk of an exposure that is usually episodic. Again, the exposure can go unnoticed. There is also a risk of infection through bite, non-bite, or aerosol routes. In these groups, primary prophylaxis is advised at the recommended dosage. Serological testing is advised every 2 years and a booster vaccination may be given if the antibody level falls below acceptable levels. The third category of people has only an infrequent risk of exposure. This group includes veterinarians and terrestrial animal-control workers in areas where rabies is uncommon to rare, veterinary students, and travelers visiting areas where rabies is enzootic and immediate access to appropriate medical care, including biologics, is limited. Just the primary prophylaxis with three injections of the vaccine is sufficient for this group. No antibody testing or routine booster vaccinations are advised for them. Other individuals living in rabies-epizootic areas do not require routine pre-exposure prophylaxis because the chance of exposure is rare.

Intradermal Injections to Save the Vaccine

The intradermal route of injection involves injecting the vaccine directly into the upper layer of skin. This method is not licensed in the United States but is used as a mode of pre-exposure prophylaxis elsewhere in the world. Only a small amount of vaccine is needed through this route. The schedule is the same as the intramuscular route: days 0, 7, and either 21 or 28. Specially packaged HDCV is used for this purpose. The injection is given directly into the skin and not underneath it. A correct vaccination should result in the formation of a tiny bleb in the skin. If this is not seen or the vaccine leaks, another injection in the other arm should be given. This method of administration requires only 0.1 mL of the vaccine instead of the 1.0 mL used through the intramuscular route. This small difference could result in huge cost savings in developing countries with poor resources. However, the vaccine meant for 1.0-mL intramuscular injections cannot be used to give multiple intradermal injections. Specially packaged intradermal vaccines should be used exclusively for this purpose. The intradermal route may result in antibody responses that are not as lasting as the intramuscular route. Antimalarial medications such as chloroquine might diminish the antibody response if taken along with the vaccine given through the intradermal route. In 1983, a Peace Corps volunteer died of rabies despite a full intradermal pre-exposure series.

Death of a Peace Corps Volunteer in Kenya after Pre-Exposure Prophylaxis

A 23-year-old Peace Corps volunteer working east of Nairobi, Kenya, was bitten by her puppy on May 31, 1983. The patient had received three intradermal doses of 0.1 mL of HDCV for pre-exposure prophylaxis (CDC, 1983b). Medical records indicated the last dose she received was in late November 1982. She was reportedly informed at that time that additional doses of vaccine would be necessary should a rabies exposure occur. In Kenya, a neighbor gave her a puppy as a gift, but failed to mention that the mother of the puppy had died of rabies, endemic in Kenya. The patient's May 31st diary entry described a behavioral change in her puppy (which was too young to be immunized against rabies) and her hope that he was not rabid. The puppy subsequently disappeared and she never learned how it had died. The patient was well until approximately August 8, when she noted pain in the left arm. On

August 10, she was seen in a Nairobi medical clinic with complaints of insomnia and increasing left arm, shoulder, and neck pain. She was hospitalized on August 11 and placed in the intensive care unit. She died of rabies on August 27, 89 days after the bite and 20 days after the onset of symptoms. CDC isolated rabies virus from a cervical cord specimen obtained at autopsy. Further testing also confirmed the diagnosis of rabies.

This was the first case of human rabies reported in a person with a history of pre-exposure rabies prophylaxis with HDCV. CDC tests showed that the vaccine had stimulated her immune system but only slightly, certainly not enough to protect her from rabies disease. CDC also checked more than 700 other Peace Corps volunteers who had also received HDCV and found that one-half responded in an immunologically weak way to the vaccine. The intradermal route of vaccine administration was suspected to be responsible for this poor immune response and the intradermal route has been discarded ever since in the United States. Another factor that can cause a poor immune response is a loss of potency of the vaccine because of the lack of refrigerating facilities and a break in the cold chain of transport. Simultaneous ingestion of chloroquine for the prophylaxis for malaria also might lessen the immune response to rabies vaccines.

Pre-exposure prophylaxis with rabies vaccine in immunocompromised individuals such as persons with AIDS (acquired immunodeficiency syndrome) might fail to induce effective antibody titers, especially with the intradermal route. Persons with impaired immunity are advised to avoid circumstances that will require vaccination. If this is impossible, the intramuscular route is preferred and the antibody titers should be checked to ensure an adequate response.

POSTEXPOSURE PROPHYLAXIS FOR RABIES

Efficient prophylaxis is available after exposure to rabies. Any wound from animals potentially carrying rabies virus should be washed thoroughly and medical attention sought. The decision to administer prophylaxis and the type of prophylaxis depends on several factors such as type of exposure, the causative animal, as well as laboratory and surveillance information for the area where the exposure occurred. Rabies is transmitted through saliva and the nervous tissue of the affected animal. If exposure has happened to either of these, an evaluation for postexposure prophylaxis (PEP) is necessary. Simple petting or handling of an animal or contact with body fluids such as blood, feces, and urine does not constitute an exposure and hence does not warrant PEP.

Type of Exposure

The type of exposure can be divided into bite and non-bite. Any penetration of the skin by the teeth of an animal constitutes a bite exposure. All bites, regardless of body site, represent a potential risk for rabies transmission. The risk varies with the species of biting animal, the anatomic site of the bite, and the severity of the wound. Bites by some animals, such as bats, can inflict minor injury that may go unnoticed. Non-bite exposures rarely cause rabies. The contamination of open wounds, abrasions, mucous membranes, or scratches with infectious material from a rabid animal constitutes a non-bite exposure.

The circumstances under which the bite occurred are also important to note. Generally, unprovoked bites carry a high risk because the animal is more likely to be rabid. Bites occurring during feeding or handling of an apparently healthy animal should be regarded as a provoked bite. Local rabies epidemiology in the area, the biting animal's history and current health status (e.g., abnormal behavior, signs of illness), and the potential for the animal to be exposed to rabies (e.g., presence of an unexplained wound or history of exposure to a rabid animal) should also be considered in deciding about PEP. The animal type greatly influences the decision to vaccinate. The current CDC guidelines are given in Table 4.1 (CDC, 2007b).

Table 4.1.
CDC Recommendations for PEP

Animal type	Evaluation and disposition of animal	PEP recommendations
Dogs, cats, and ferrets	Healthy and available for 10 day observation	Persons should not begin vaccination unless animal develops clinical signs of rabies
	Rabid or suspected rabid	Immediately vaccinate
	Unknown (escaped)	Consult public health officials
Raccoons, skunks, foxes, and most other carnivores; bats	Regarded as rabid unless animal is proven negative by laboratory tests	Consider immediate vaccination
Livestock, horses, rodents, rabbits and hares, and other mammals	Consider individually	Consult public health officials
		Bites of squirrels, hamsters, guinea pigs, gerbils, chipmunks, rats, mice, other small rodents, rabbits, and hares almost never require rabies PEP

More cats than dogs developed rabies during the years 2000–2004. This could be due to the spillover effect of the raccoon rabies epidemic of the East Coast. Alternatively, lack of cat vaccination or leash laws and the curiosity and roaming habits of cats might also place cats at a higher risk of contracting the disease. Exposure to any other domestic animal should be conveyed to the public health authorities before a decision to euthanize the animal is taken. Exotic pets kept in homes should be considered the same as other wild animals. The current vaccines are not licensed to be used in these situations, but an off-label use is possible. Moreover, simple observation is not advisable because the nature of virus shedding in these species is unknown and erratic. Just the fact that the animal is healthy at day 10 does not mean that the animal did not have rabies.

Other Wild Animals

All bites by wild animals such as raccoons, skunks, foxes, and coyotes should be considered a possible exposure to the rabies virus. These are the terrestrial animals most often infected with rabies in the United States. PEP should begin as soon as possible following exposure to such wildlife unless the animal has already been tested and determined not to be rabid. If the animal is subsequently tested as negative for rabies, the PEP can be discontinued at that time. Signs of rabies among wildlife cannot be interpreted reliably; therefore, any such animal that exposes a person should be euthanized as soon as possible (without unnecessary damage to the head) and the brain should be submitted for rabies testing. If the results of the testing are negative, PEP can be discontinued.

Other wild animals such as small rodents (e.g., squirrels, hamsters, guinea pigs, gerbils, chipmunks, rats, and mice) and lagomorphs (including rabbits and hares) are almost never found to be infected with rabies and have not been known to transmit rabies to humans. From 1990 through 1996, in areas of the United States where raccoon rabies was common, woodchucks (groundhogs) accounted for 93 percent of the 371 cases of rabies among rodents reported to the CDC. In all cases involving rodents, the state or local health department should be consulted before starting PEP. The offspring of wild animals crossbred to domestic dogs and cats (wild animal hybrids) are considered wild animals. Wild animals and wild animal hybrids should not be kept as pets. In instances in which wild or hybrid animals are suspected of rabies, they should be euthanized and tested for rabies.

Avoid Contact with Wild Animals

Rabies prevention also can be achieved by minimizing the interaction of any wildlife and humans or pets in general. Wild animals usually visit human habitats with the purpose of finding food and shelter. The preventive efforts can be started by inspecting the property and removing any sites that could be used by wild animals for sleeping or raising their young. This can be especially useful in rural areas or isolated households. Chimneys should be capped and all of the holes in the roofs, eaves, and the side of the building should be sealed. Tree limbs extending over the roof should be trimmed to prevent access. Bright exterior lighting will discourage wild animals. If there is a wild animal problem, the entire neighborhood should adopt these measures so that the neighborhood is not wild-animal friendly.

The house and the yard should be free of food. Animal-proof lids can be used for garbage cans and they should be stored in a secure place. Feeding of pets outside is not a good idea because food remnants may be left, attracting wild animals. Gardens could also attract wildlife such as raccoons. A low-voltage electric fence is a viable option. A two-wire fence, with one wire 4–6 inches above the ground and the other at 12 inches, is usually effective. A humane live trap is another option. Raccoons can be baited with several foods because they will eat virtually anything. If a raccoon is trapped, the animal should be handled carefully and released at least 3 miles away.

If an animal is already raising young in the vicinity of a household, it is advisable to wait until the young leave the den. When the young ones are gone, the entrance to the den can be blocked after the animals have left for the night. Alternatively, flaps opening only to one side can be used if the entrance cannot be watched. The animals will be able to leave the den by raising the lid but are unable to re-enter because they cannot push back the flap. A bright light directly shining into the den or a loud radio on all day also might discourage the animal from returning. If the animal is persistent, the local animal control officer should be called.

Animal Observation

In North America, a healthy dog, cat, or ferret that bites an individual can be observed for 10 days for the signs and symptoms of rabies. If the animal does not develop the features of rabies within 10 days, it may be presumed that the animal is not shedding the virus at the time of the bite. This is based on the observation that these animals always develop rabies within 10 days of shedding the virus in the saliva. Recent observations in ferrets confirm the utility of this strategy (Jackson and Wunner, 2002, 411). This can alleviate the use of expensive PEP measures.

Any illness in the animal during the confinement period or before release should be evaluated by a veterinarian and reported immediately to the local public health department. If signs suggestive of rabies develop, PEP should be initiated in the victims and the animal should be euthanized, with its head sent to a qualified laboratory for analysis. If the biting animal is stray or unwanted, it should either be confined and observed for 10 days or be euthanized immediately and submitted for rabies examination. Skunks, raccoons, foxes, and bats that bite humans should be euthanized and tested. Observation is not advised in these species because the length of time between the rabies virus appearing in their saliva and the onset of symptoms is unknown.

After exposure to wildlife in which rabies is suspected, prophylaxis is warranted in most circumstances. Wild animal hybrids should be euthanized and tested rather than confined and observed when they bite humans because the period of rabies virus shedding in these animals is unknown (CDC, 2007b). Vaccination should be discontinued if tests of the involved animal are negative for rabies infection.

Although rabies virus has been isolated from the human saliva, direct human-to-human transmission is extremely rare. Six anecdotal reports of human-to-human rabies transmission have been published. Medical staff caring for rabies patients do not require PEP unless there is a bite from the patient, or contact with the patient's saliva, respiratory secretions, corneas (tears), or cerebrospinal fluid with an open wound or mucous membrane.

Wound Classification and the Use of Immune Globulin (Serum)

If the wound inflicted by the biting animal is significant, large amounts of the virus can be inoculated and the risk of developing rabies is higher and faster. Because of this reason, simultaneous administration of the immune globulin is advised. The antibody response caused by the virus will take some time before it is effective. The idea is to administer those antibodies taken from another individual directly to the patient at the time of starting the vaccination. There are problems in universally choosing this strategy. The immune globulin used for this purpose is costly and not easily available. This is produced from vaccinated individuals so it has all of the potential complications of blood products, such as the transmission of other infections and unusual reactions.

The wound care should start with immediate cleansing and flushing of the wound with soap and water or water alone and disinfection with ethanol or tincture of iodine. Proper wound care is the first line of defense against rabies. Washing of the wound might help to reduce rabies virus infection by eliminating or inactivating the virus particles inoculated in the tissue at the time of the animal bite. Primary closure of the wound by suturing should be avoided as much as possible. Other general measures such as tetanus prophylaxis and

Table 4.2.
WHO Classification of Animal Bite Wounds

Category of wound	Type of contact/bite	Recommendations
Category I	Touching, feeding of animals or licks on intact skin	No treatment if history is reliable
Category II	Minor scratches or abrasions without bleeding or licks on broken skin and nibbling of uncovered skin	Use vaccine alone
Category III	Single or multiple transdermal bites, scratches or contamination of mucous membrane with saliva (i.e., licks)	Use immune globulin (serum) plus vaccine

antibiotic treatment may be indicated in appropriate circumstances, especially in wounds associated with significant tissue damage. If surgical manipulation is inevitable, rabies immune globulin should be given before the procedure.

Initiation of specific treatment should not await the results of laboratory diagnosis or be delayed by dog observation when rabies is suspected. Pregnancy and infancy are never contraindications to rabies postexposure treatment. Persons who present for evaluation and treatment even months after having been bitten should be dealt with in the same manner as if the contact occurred recently. WHO has classified the bite wounds into three categories for the purpose of determining the treatment course for the PEP (WHO, 2002).

Human Rabies Immune Globulin

The human rabies immune globulin (HRIG) is prepared from healthy volunteers immunized with the rabies vaccine. The antibodies that are formed against rabies are purified. There are two products available in the U.S. market. Imogam® is a sterile solution of HRIG (10–18 percent protein) for intramuscular administration manufactured by Aventis Pasteur SA. It is prepared by cold alcohol fractionation from pooled venous plasma of individuals immunized with rabies vaccine prepared from human diploid cells. The other product is called HyperRab®, manufactured by Talecris Biotherapeutics, Inc. This product is also prepared by cold ethanol fractionation of immune globulins from the plasma of donors hyperimmunized with rabies vaccine. Both are indicated for intramuscular injection as a part of the PEP in category III wounds. Rabies antibody provides immediate passive protection when given to individuals exposed to the rabies virus. Immune globulins are derived from human plasma. Products made from human plasma may contain infectious agents, such as viruses, that can cause disease. The risk of this occurrence has been reduced by screening plasma donors for prior exposure to certain viruses, by testing for the presence of certain current virus infections, and by inactivating and/or removing certain viruses (Rupprecht and Gibbons, 2004).

HRIG should never be administered in the same syringe or into the same anatomical site as the rabies vaccine. Simultaneous administration might result in interference with the potency of the vaccine. Because HRIG may partially suppress active production of antibody, no more than the recommended dose should be given. Certain vaccinations, such as the measles vaccination, should be deferred if a patient has recently received rabies immune globulin because of the chance of interference with the immunological response. HRIG should be given to a pregnant woman only if clearly needed. The side effects of the immune globulins include headaches, other systemic symptoms such as malaise, and local adverse reactions such as tenderness, pain, soreness or stiffness of the muscles at the injection site. These symptoms may be treated symptomatically. Although not reported specifically for HRIG, angioneurotic edema, nephrotic syndrome, and anaphylaxis have been reported after injection of immune globulin (Ig), a product similar in biochemical composition but without antirabies activity. Ig is a sterilized solution obtained from pooled human blood plasma obtained from normal healthy volunteers. These volunteers are not deliberately immunized against any infectious agents including rabies. Ig contains immunoglobulins (or antibodies) to protect against several infectious agents that cause various diseases; however, rabies is not one of them.

PEP in Nonimmunized Patients

PEP differs slightly depending upon the individual's prior rabies vaccination status. A previously nonimmunized individual will require more doses of the vaccine (usually five) for PEP. One milliliter of human diploid cell vaccine (HDCV) or the purified chick embryo cell vaccine (PCECV) is given intramuscularly on days 0, 3, 7, 14, and 28 (CDC, 1999). The first dose of the five-dose course should be administered as soon as possible after exposure. For adults, the vaccination should always be administered in the deltoid area (upper arm). The anterolateral aspect of the thigh is also acceptable in children. The gluteal area should never be used for rabies vaccine injections because observations suggest administration in this area results in lower neutralizing antibody titers.

Category III wounds also require HRIG administration (WHO, 2002). The recommended dose of HRIG is 20 IU/kg body weight. This formula is applicable to all age groups, including children. If possible, the full dose should be infiltrated around any wound(s) and any remaining volume should be administered intramuscularly at an anatomical site distant from vaccine administration. HRIG should not be administered in the same syringe as vaccine. HRIG may be diluted with saline if the volume is not adequate to infiltrate around all wounds. Equine rabies immune globulin is available outside North America. This rabies immune globulin is produced from horses that are hyperimmunized with the rabies vaccine. Because of the animal origin, this product has more complications including serious reactions such as anaphylaxis and serum sickness. The dose is 40 mL/kg and may be administered the same way as HRIG (Jackson and Wunner, 2002, 413). The equine rabies immune globulin is widely used in developing countries because of its lower cost and greater availability.

PEP for Previously Immunized Individuals

In previously immunized individuals, two intramuscular doses (1.0 mL each) of the rabies vaccine, one immediately and one 3 days later, is sufficient. Previously vaccinated persons are those who have received one of the recommended pre-exposure or postexposure regimens of HDCV, RVA, or PCECV, or those who have received another vaccine and had a documented rabies antibody titer. Rabies immune globulin is unnecessary and should not be administered to these persons because an anamnestic response will follow the administration of a booster regardless of the pre-booster antibody titer. The rabies immune globulin can actually hinder this response.

Postexposure Treatment in Immunocompromised Individuals

As in the case of pre-exposure prophylaxis, the rabies vaccines might not stimulate adequate immunological response in immunocompromised individuals such as those with AIDS. This is also related to the lymphocyte count in the blood. Because of these facts, the most effective regimen in immunocompromised patients after an exposure is thorough wound care using soap, water, and povidone iodine followed by administration of the rabies immune globulin. The rabies immune globulin can be used with the same protocol as described for immunocompetent individuals. All immunocompromised patients with category II and III wounds should receive rabies immune globulin as well as five doses of vaccine.

Shortened Regimens of Postexposure Treatment

WHO has advised using a shortened version of the vaccination, given through the intramuscular route, to save the amount of vaccine used,

especially in developing countries. One of these regimens is known as 2–1–
1.The numbers indicate the number of vaccine shots on each day. In the 2–1–
1 schedule, two doses of vaccine are given in each upper arm on day 0. A single dose is repeated on day 7 and another on day 21. The injections can be
given in alternate upper arms. Thai researchers have formulated an alternative
intradermal treatment for postexposure treatment to save the amount of vaccine. This schedule is known as 8–0–4–0–1–1. This consists of injecting eight
sites intradermally with 0.1 mL on day 0, no vaccine on day 3, four sites on
day 7, no vaccine on day 14, and one site each on days 28 and 90 (Jackson
and Wunner, 2002, 417).

Pregnancy

Pregnancy is not a contraindication for postexposure treatment. A few studies in which pregnant patients received rabies vaccine and immunoglobulin
showed no major untoward effects. One study revealed eight (4.2 percent)
spontaneous abortions. This abortion rate was thought to be similar to the
general population. Alternatively, trauma from the dog bite might also have
contributed to the spontaneous abortions (Jackson and Wunner 2002, 417).

PEP in Developing Countries

Most of the cases of rabies deaths occur in developing countries. It is
believed that more than 20,000 patients die every year from rabies in India.
The actual numbers may be higher because of poor reporting and inadequate
facilities for accurate diagnosis. Worldwide, several countries where rabies is
endemic do not even have a reporting program. Canine rabies is the most
common culprit in all of these areas, compounded by the problems of stray
dogs. If the vaccination rates in the dog population are more than 70 percent,
then 96.5 percent of all the major outbreaks of rabies will be prevented. This
goal is unattainable because of poor resources, lack of motivation, and low
awareness. Another problem developing countries are facing is the affordability of the advanced cell culture vaccines that are much safer, more effective,
and acceptable to patients. Neural tissue-derived vaccines are still used in several areas. For example, two-thirds of the 3 million patients who receive rabies
postexposure treatment in India every year receive the Semple vaccine, which
is a neural tissue-derived vaccine, with high incidence of neuroparalytic complications. A concerted effort by world and regional government authorities,
vaccine manufacturers, and non-governmental agencies is the only way to rectify this situation.

PREVENTING RABIES FROM BATS

Bats pose interesting problems in rabies PEP. In the United States, rabid bats have been documented in all 50 states except Hawaii. Bats are increasingly becoming the most important wildlife reservoir for rabies in the United States. Minor, seemingly unimportant, or unrecognized bites from bats can cause rabies transmission. Any bat that is active by day, found in a place where bats are not usually seen, (e.g., in a room in the house or on the lawn), or is unable to fly should be suspected to be suffering from rabies. An untrained person should never handle bats and they should never be kept as pets. If there is a question of bat exposure, the bat should be safely collected and submitted for rabies diagnosis. It is also important to remember that people cannot get rabies from having contact with bat guano (feces), blood, or urine; from touching a bat on its fur; or seeing a bat in an attic, in a cave, or from a distance. If a bat bites a person or if infectious material (such as saliva) from a bat gets into the eyes, nose, mouth, or a wound, the affected area should be thoroughly washed and medical attention should be sought immediately. Whenever possible, the bat responsible should be captured and sent to a laboratory for rabies testing. The local public health department can assist with this. Rabies can only be confirmed in a laboratory, but is very probable in bats showing unusual behavior.

Rabies PEP is recommended for all persons with bite, scratch, or mucous membrane exposure to a bat, unless the bat is available for testing and is negative for evidence of rabies. PEP should be considered when direct contact between a human and a bat has occurred, unless the exposed person can be certain a bite, scratch, or mucous membrane exposure did not occur. If a bat is found indoors and there is no history of bat-human contact, the likely effectiveness of PEP must be balanced against the low risk of such exposures. PEP should be considered for persons who were in the same room as a bat who might be unaware that a bite or direct contact has occurred if rabies cannot be ruled out by testing the bat. If a sleeping person awakens to find a bat in the room, or an adult witnesses a bat in the room with a previously unattended child, mentally disabled person, or intoxicated person, this qualifies for PEP. PEP is not warranted for other household members in these situations.

Facts about Bats

Control of bats, prevention of their entry to human habitat, and minimizing their contact with humans are main methods of rabies control, especially in North America. This is very important in light of increased recognition of rabies among bats and the emergence of bats as the premier rabies-carrying species. Bats belong to a group of their own, called *Chiroptera*, meaning "hand-wing" (Bat Conservation International, 2008). Bats are very unique in that they are the only flying mammals in the world. Contrary to popular belief, bats are not blind. They use "echolocation" to determine their surroundings and navigate while flying. Bats are the most successful predators of night-flying insects. Seventy percent of bat species survive on insects. Some bats can consume as many as 600 mosquitoes in an hour. Several tropical species feed exclusively on fruit or nectar. A few other bat species are mainly carnivores, hunting for small animals such as fish, reptiles, mice, and birds. A single bat can eat up to 3,000 insects in one night and an average-size colony can eat up to a half million insects every night. In temperate regions, bats hibernate during the cold winters. They migrate up to 300 miles to find a suitable cave or abandoned mine. They can live 6 months or more depending solely upon their stored fat reserves. Hibernation is a state of prolonged inactivity during which bats greatly reduce their normal metabolic activities. Their body temperature falls from a normal level of more than 100°F to that of the surrounding cave temperature, usually 40–50°F. The heart rate slows to about 20 beats per minute, in contrast to 1,000 beats per minute during flight. Hibernating bats survive on a very small amount of stored fat during the 5- to 6-month period, conserving a significant amount of energy. They might lose 25–50 percent of their prehibernation body weight.

Bats have important ecological functions including pollination, seed dispersion, especially in the tropics, and decreasing the insect population such as mosquitoes. Bats are the major predator of night-flying insects, including pests that cost farmers billions of dollars annually. Not all bats are dangerous. Less than 0.5 percent of bats actually carry rabies. Bats flying erratically during the daytime might indicate disease. They should not be approached or handled because their defensive response will likely be to bite the individual.

Bats are widely misunderstood creatures worldwide. They are perceived as shady, frightening creatures because of their nocturnal habits and unusual practices, such as roosting upside down. Bats are closely associated with Halloween as scary creatures. In the Philippines, 1.8 million fruit bats roost in a cave on the island of Samal. They come out of the cave in a stream, undulating against a red sunset. They look like a shadowy cloud in the sky at dusk. These bats help the local economy significantly by performing the pollination of the durian trees (fruit popular in East Asia). They also ingest millions of pests that can damage the local crops, but local farmers think that they are responsible for the loss of coffee crops and try to kill the bats. However the fact is that bats do not eat coffee, but only other overripe fruits that will waste anyway. Killing the bats is not only unnecessary, but actually harmful to the farming economy.

Bats can squeeze through the tiniest of openings because of their body contour. They can crawl through crevices as small as 5/8 inch. Bats can gain entry to buildings through a variety of locations; the wrong type of caulk or sealant can aggravate this problem. Bats typically use chimneys to gain entry into a house. Other vulnerable areas include loose or missing sidings, outside facing vents, fatigued screens, degraded wood, gaps in log homes, and gaps between trim boards or exterior walls. Most bats roost in secluded locations away from humans, but some species such as the little brown bat and the big brown bat in the northeastern United States repeatedly roost in attics. Traditionally, their roosting place was in hollow trees, but they adapted to roost in houses after early settlers eliminated vast expanses of forests. They also like to roost in attics because hot attics act as incubators for young and growing pups.

Bat-Proofing

Bat-proofing a building involves sealing all entrance holes so that bats cannot enter into the house. There are several professional services available for this purpose. Bat-proofing could also be a "do-it-yourself" project. Diligently identifying the entrances used by bats is the first step towards bat-proofing. The holes that bats use to enter or exit an attic must be carefully located. Bats commonly enter at points where joined materials have warped, shrunk, or pulled away from each other, leaving tiny gaps. Vents with loose screening, roof peaks, and roof or siding joints are some of the favored points of entry by bats. The presence of telltale bat droppings will give clues to the site of entry. Inspection from inside the attic can reveal openings preferred by bats. If a

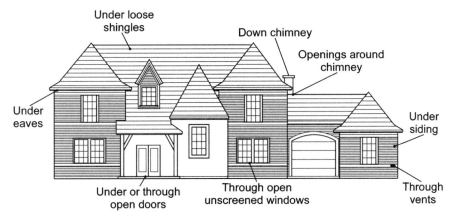

Common bat entry points in a house. (CDC, 2006. Redrawn by Jeff Dixon)

person enters the attic, the bats will quickly retreat out of sight rather than take flight. So if bats are not seen right away, listen for the squeaking or scurrying sounds that will verify their presence. Bat droppings seen inside will also indicate entry routes. With attic lights turned off during the day, points of outside light seeping into the attic will be revealed. These are the same entry points used by bats to gain access to the house; hence, sealing them will help bat-proof the house.

Staging a "bat watch" is also helpful in determining the entry points of bats. At dusk, two persons can wait at the two sides of the building and watch for any bats leaving the house. Once bats are seen exiting from the house, watch that area of the house for more bats. Dawn is another excellent time to detect the entry points. The returning bats will swarm around the entrance a few times before actually entering the house.

Sealing Entrances

Once the bat entrances have been located, the next step in bat-proofing is to seal these entry points. Because bats can crawl through astonishingly small crevices, any openings larger than 0.25 by 0.5 inches should be caulked. Loosely hanging clear plastic sheeting or bird netting over those areas at dusk may initially be the best strategy. This will exclude the bats from coming back. However, this will not prevent any remaining bats in the house from crawling out and leaving through the lower part of such materials. Window screening or hardware cloth can be used to cover louvered vents or large gaps and cracks in the building. After the bats have been excluded, expanding foam insulation or caulking can be used to seal small crevices. After proper hardening, this can be trimmed or painted. Bats will not gnaw new holes in the building unlike mice, and proper sealing will help to exclude the bats from coming back to the house. Chimney caps and draft-guards beneath doors can also be used for this purpose. All electrical and plumbing holes should be sealed with appropriate materials, and all doors to the outside should close tightly. Most bat-proofing materials can be obtained at local hardware or building supply stores.

Timing of Bat-Proofing

Timing is important for bat-proofing because of the habit of hibernation among bats. During summer, many young bats are unable to fly. If adult bats are excluded during this time, the young ones may be trapped inside the home and may die. Alternatively, they can also make their way into other parts of the house. Female bats may try frantically to re-enter the house even during daylight hours to rejoin their young ones. It is best to avoid bat-proofing between the months of May and August. Most bats leave their habitats in the fall or winter for hibernation. The best time for bat-proofing a home is in the spring, before bats enter the roost, or in the fall, after the bats have left.

Big brown bats occasionally sleep through the winter in a building by hibernating in the attic or basement. Installing a one-way door in the fall, before the bats begin hibernating, or in the spring, before the pups are born, is the best way to bat-proof the home in this situation. Whenever bats are suspected to inhabit a building, the best way to bat-proof is to install a one-way door. They are designed to allow the bats to leave but not to enter. One-way doors are pieces of mesh or screening placed over a bat entrance to form a long sleeve or tent. Bats will exit at night through the bottom but the door will prevent their reentry at dawn. These types of doors work because bats determine the entrance of their habitat by the use of smell and not by their vision. On return they will land on the mesh and focus on the entrance hole and the mesh will not let them in. Bats will not move to the opening at the bottom of the door to gain entrance. A schedule for bat-proofing without endangering them is given below.

- January–April: Seal entrances before bats return to the building.
- May–August: Watch bats to identify entrances. Do not seal openings.
- August–October: Install one-way door(s).
- November–December: Seal entrances once bats have left the building. (If bats are suspected to be hibernating in the building, install a one-way door during September–October).

Installing One-Way Doors

Installing one-way doors can be done by choosing a 0.25- to 0.5-inch wire screening or heavy plastic mesh to cover the bats' point of entry. The screening should be cut so that it covers the width of the hole and extends approximately 3 feet below the hole. The screening should project 3–5 inches clear of the hole so that the bats can crawl between the screen and the building and exit at the bottom. The mesh can be secured at the top and sides with duct tape or staples and leave the bottom open. The door should be left at least 3–4 days, until it is definite that all the bats have left the building. The opening can be permanently sealed afterwards. Avoid one-way doors during the months of May–August to avoid trapping the young ones.

Catching a Single Bat at Home

There are primarily two scenarios in which humans and bats find themselves in conflict: (1) when a lone bat flies into a building, or (2) when a maternity colony of bats roosts in a building. Individual bats occasionally wander and enter houses, most often during summer evenings. These wayward bats are usually young pups that are just beginning to fly. A bat trapped in a house will usually fly in circles looking for an exit. Penn State College of Agricultural Sciences provides detailed directions in their booklet, *Home Owners Guide to North Eastern Bats and Bat Problems* (Williams and Brittingham, 2006, 5–6). The best method for getting a bat out of the house is to allow it to find its own way out. Chasing or swatting at the bat should be avoided because it may cause the bat to panic and fly erratically around the room. All doors leading to other rooms in the house should be shut to confine the bat to as small an area as possible. All windows and doors opening to the outside should be opened to give the bat a chance to escape. Any pets should be removed from the room. Leave the lights on and stand quietly against the wall or the door and watch the bat until it leaves the room. Instead of herding the bat towards an open window, the bat should be allowed to find its own way outside through the window. Bats usually make steep banking turns indoors. They fly upwards near a wall and swoop lower near the center of the room. Usually within 10–15 minutes, the bat will locate a window or door to the outside and leave.

If the bat tires and comes to rest on a curtain or wall, it can be easily removed without directly touching it. The following steps can be adopted, but one should remember never to touch the bat with bare hands.

1. Put on a pair of leather gardening or work gloves to avoid direct skin contact with the bat. If possible, wear a face shield to protect contact with mucous membranes (eyes, nose, and mouth) or skin contact around the head and neck.
2. Place a container, such as a large plastic bowl, over the bat as it rests on the wall. At this point, the bat is probably exhausted, disoriented, and will not fly as you approach it. (If it does take flight, stand back and follow the procedure for flying out bats as described previously.)
3. Slide a piece of rigid cardboard between the container and the wall to trap the bat. Hold the cardboard firmly against the container and carry the container outside.
4. Place the container (facing away from you) on a secure place above the ground (such as on a ledge, or against a tree) and slide away the cardboard. The bat will not fly right away, so releasing it above the ground keeps it safe from predators until it has its bearings. Unlike birds, most bats must drop from a perch and catch air under their wings before they can fly.

If there are recurring problems with bats entering the home, the attic should be inspected to determine the presence of a bat maternity colony. If the building is housing a bat maternity colony, follow the steps to bat-proof the house. The attic can also be inspected for bat droppings during the night. The dry, black droppings are about the size of a grain of rice and accumulate in piles below areas where the bats roost. This should be differentiated from mouse droppings, which are usually scattered in small amounts throughout the attic. Bats living in the attic during the day and large accumulations of bat droppings suggest a maternity bat colony in the house.

If a bat is suspected to be rabid or has inflicted injury to an individual, the animal can be caught using the same techniques already described. It is important to avoid trauma to the head of the animal because it is needed for the rabies test. Do not use a glue board to capture the animal because the bat then cannot be easily removed for rabies testing. Gloves used in capture should be sprayed or wiped with a bleach/water mixture (1 cup bleach to 1 gallon water) or a disinfectant solution, or disposed. If a bat is not within arms reach, an extension pole with a net may be used to capture it. While wearing gloves (heavy, preferably pliable thick leather), slowly approach the bat with a net and rotate the pole so that the bat is scooped into the net. By turning the net, the bat will be captured inside. A gloved hand can be used to grab the bat through the outside of the net. Next, a coffee can is slid into the net, pushing the bat into the can. The lid or a piece of cardboard is placed on the can to contain the bat. If there is a delay of more than 4 hours before the rabies testing of the captured bat, the canned bat should be bagged in plastic and placed in a cooler or refrigerated area. A bat should not be stored in the same cooler or refrigerator as food. The specimen also should be kept away from potential contact with people or other animals. The canned bat is labeled with the date of capture, location, and the name of exposed individual.

A total of 299 bat incidents were reported at 109 children's camps in New York from 1998 to 2002; 1,429 campers and staff were involved, and 461 persons received rabies treatment. In 53.8 percent of the incidents, the bat was captured and samples tested negative for rabies virus. Altogether 61.3 percent of persons did not receive any rabies prophylaxis (Robbins A, et al., 2005) CDC suggests the following general measures to reduce the risk of contracting rabies.

1. Teach children never to handle unfamiliar animals, wild or domestic, even if they appear friendly. "Love your own, leave other animals alone" is a good principle for children to learn.
2. Wash any wound from an animal thoroughly with soap and water and seek medical attention immediately.

3. Have all dead, sick, or easily captured bats tested for rabies if exposure to people or pets occurs.

4. Prevent bats from entering living quarters or occupied spaces in homes, churches, schools, and other similar areas where they might come into contact with people and pets.

5. Be a responsible pet owner by keeping vaccinations up to date for all dogs, cats, and ferrets. Keep cats and ferrets inside and dogs under direct supervision, call animal control to remove stray animals from the neighborhood, and consider having pets spayed or neutered (CDC, 2007c).

What If a Pet is Bitten by a Bat?

Whenever a dog, cat, or other domestic animal with up-to-date rabies vaccinations is bitten by or comes into contact with a bat, the bat should be captured if possible. The methods previously explained will help in accomplishing this task safely. Testing the bat for rabies should be arranged immediately with the local health authority. If the bat is rabid or is not available for testing, the animal must be given a rabies booster vaccination within 5 days. If an unvaccinated animal has contact with a rabid or suspected rabid bat, the animal must be quarantined for 6 months or humanely euthanized.

Bats in the Caves

During hibernation, bats survive without eating by slowly metabolizing stored fat. To conserve their fat resources, bats drastically lower their metabolic rate and enter a state of deep sleep. Caving, also called spelunking, is the recreational sport of exploring caves. When people enter a cave, their lights, voices, and body heat disturb the bats' sleep, often to the point where they awake completely and take flight. It is estimated that a bat can burn 10–30 days worth of stored fat reserves during each of these awakenings. If this happens too many times over the course of a winter, the bats may starve to death before spring or leave the cave in such a weakened condition that they cannot successfully reproduce. Recreational cavers can prevent disturbing bats by avoiding trips to recreational and commercial caves during the hibernation season (December through March). When cavers do encounter hibernating bats, they should leave the cave quickly and quietly, taking care not to shine their lights on the sleeping bats. Fortunately, most spelunkers are very considerate of bats and have found ways to minimize their impact on bats and cave environments.

Vampire Bat Control Methods

Measures to control vampire bat rabies include efforts to prevent bat bites, pre-exposure rabies prophylaxis for animals (cattle) and humans at risk (e.g., bat workers, control operators, and vets), and PEP for people who are bitten. Destruction of bats in the wild, both in their natural habitat and in the vicinity of livestock, is also found to be helpful. In cattle, prophylactic vaccination for rabies is very effective with some vaccines offering protection up to 100 percent. The cost of the vaccine and the willingness of the cattle farmers are the major barriers to this strategy.

Reduction of vampire bat populations can be achieved either by the destruction of bats in their wild environment or by poisoning them in the vicinity of cattle where they usually hover. Vampire bats have a low reproductive potential with a gestational period of 7 months, leading to the birth of a single offspring. Techniques used to control vampire bats are the use of firearms with scatter-shot cartridges, electrocution of bats in caves, and the usage of smoke and fire to drive bats from hollow trees and caves. Other substances such as dynamite, gasoline bombs, and poison gas—especially Rhodiatrox (a phosphorus-based compound) and cyanide gas—are also used to drive bats out. Biological methods have also been used to control vampire bats. In Columbia, 5,000 vampire bats were destroyed by infecting them with Newcastle disease virus via airborne instillation of atomized virus. This method of indiscriminate killing of bats could become dangerous to the human population and other animals. All of these methods share the disadvantage of being nonselective. During the Second World War, United States armed forces used flamethrowers in the Caribbean island of Trinidad to exterminate vampire bats abundant in that country's caves. This method was discontinued as dangerous and not practical. Smoke and fire must be used with extreme caution because hollow trees can catch fire. Several other useful types of bats may roost with the vampire bats. Needless destruction of these bats might have far reaching ecological and agricultural consequences.

Other methods have targeted bats while they are in the process of attacking cattle. Poisons such as strychnine and arsenic and various anticoagulants have been used for this purpose. Poisons can be directly applied to wounds because vampire bats tend to return to the previous wounds they have inflicted. The serious drawback of these poisons is the health risks posed to the workers who apply them. Vampire bats are very sensitive to anticoagulants (substances that prevent coagulation or clotting and thus cause uncontrolled bleeding). Anticoagulants such as diphenadione can be injected to cattle in doses that will not harm them. When the bats feast on these cattle, they are killed because of the effects of these anticoagulants. This method is usually effective only for a short period of time (i.e., 3 days) and necessitates frequent injections to the cattle. Potential toxicity to calves is another concern. Intramuscular administration of warfarin, the common rat poison, is also effective in controlling the bats, and this is easier to administer.

Anticoagulants may also be applied directly to vampire bats in their roosts and will rapidly spread through the colony by mutual grooming. However, this process can kill other species of bats that are beneficial, so this method has been discontinued. Anticoagulants may also be applied directly, in the form of a paste, to the open wounds of cattle.

Various other species of bats have also been affected by these vampire bat extermination campaigns. An estimated 900,000 bats of various species were gassed annually in Venezuela from 1964 to 1966. In Mexico, entrances of caves were barricaded with chicken wire in the belief that vampire bats were roosting inside, resulting in the death of several bat species. The deleterious effects of burning hollow trees to exterminate bats have been mentioned already. The potentially damaging effect on tropical ecosystems of these types of campaigns needs to be appreciated. Many bats play a crucial role in tropical ecosystems and their wholesale loss could have far reaching effects. Although reducing vampire populations may be acceptable in certain areas, the aim should not be to completely eradicate the species. In 1968, Greenhall stressed that the two major aims of vampire control should be control of the population levels of the offending species, rather than indiscriminate destruction of individuals and protection of nontarget species (Greenhall, 1968).

5

Treatment of Rabies

What happened to the 12-year-old girl from the developing country in Asia or Africa? She was diagnosed to have rabies on the basis of the clinical features. Blood tests and other sophisticated tests were not available. The physicians observed the patient closely. She became agitated at times. She was sedated. Intravenous fluids were given. Her consciousness fluctuated. She had copious secretions coming from the mouth. Her family waited anxiously. They knew the results. After an agonizing few days, she slipped into a coma and died.

Despite our remarkable advances in the treatment of infectious diseases, there is still no specific treatment for rabies. Viral diseases are difficult to treat for several reasons. To begin with, they are difficult to diagnose and often adopt a stealth mode of operation to infect the host cell. Viruses use the cells' own machinery to replicate. Any attempt to kill the virus invariably results in killing the cell as well; hence the difficulties in finding a cure for viral diseases.

The best strategy to conquer rabies is preventive therapy. The current recommendations of wound cleansing, immunization with a cell cultured vaccine, and administration of human rabies immune globulin is highly effective in the prevention of the disease. There is no role for rabies immunization once the disease manifests. At this point the rabies virus has infected the brain of the victim and the vaccine is useless.

RABIES SURVIVORS

There have been six survivors of the disease in the published scientific literature so far. All of them except the recent case from Wisconsin received some form of rabies prophylaxis (either rabies vaccine or immune globulin) prior to the onset of the illness. This might have modified the course of the disease in these patients.

First Rabies Survivor—Ohio 1971

The first recorded case of rabies survival was reported from Ohio (Hattwick MAW, et al., 1972). Matthew Winkler, a 6-year-old boy from Willshire, Ohio, battled the disease for 2 months and at the end survived miraculously without any sequelae. His ordeal began on October 10, 1970, when a bat flew into the sleeping child's bedroom and bit his left thumb. Tests done on the dead bat confirmed that it was rabid. Matthew was given a series of injections comprising a vaccine that was produced from duck embryo cell culture (PCECV). Usually this vaccine should prevent the disease if given early in the disease. However, the efforts failed. After several weeks of painful injections of a large amount of serum into the abdominal wall, Matthew became symptomatic. He complained of muscle stiffness around the neck and dizziness towards the end of October. His illness progressed and by early November he developed difficulty in speaking and moving the left arm (the arm bitten by the bat). He developed a stiff neck and the cerebrospinal fluid obtained through a lumbar puncture was abnormal. It showed a high white cell count at 125 and slightly elevated protein. These tests were not diagnostic of rabies, but Matthew later showed abnormal behavior and slipped into a coma.

He was admitted to the intensive care unit and was assisted for breathing through a respirator. A brain biopsy was consistent with encephalitis. Other tests including the blood tests showed evidence of rabies. He developed seizures and further cardiac and respiratory complications. Subsequently, his condition improved and the doctors were able to disconnect him from the ventilator. He had difficulties in walking and speaking, but with several months of therapy, made a complete recovery.

Argentina—Rabies Recovery

The second case was reported from Argentina in South America (Porras C, et al., 1976). A dog bit a 45-year-old woman multiple times on the left arm.

Table 5.1.
Human Rabies Survivors

Year	Country	Age	Sex	Mode of transmission	Immunization received	Outcome	Reference
1970	United States	6	Male	Bat bite	Duck embryo vaccine	Complete recovery	Hattwick MAW, et al., 1972.
1972	Argentina	45	Female	Dog bite	Suckling mouse brain vaccine	Minor sequelae	Porras C, et al., 1976.
1977	United States	32	Male	Laboratory vaccine strain	Duck embryo Vaccine	Sequelae	Tillotson JR, et al., 1977.
1992	Mexico	9	Male	Dog bite	Vero cell vaccine and immune globulin	Severe sequelae	Alvarez L, et al., 1994.
2002	India	6	Female	Dog bite	Chick embryo vaccine	Sequelae	Madhusudana SN, et al., 2002.
2004	United States	15	Female	Bat bite	None	Minor sequelae	Willoughby RE, et al., 2005.

The dog developed rabies and died 4 days later. The patient received a 14-day course of suckling mouse brain vaccine followed by two booster doses. Approximately 3 weeks after the bite, the patient complained of paresthesias of the arm that slowly progressed to generalized weakness. The patient was admitted to the hospital with paralysis of all four limbs. She also exhibited several neurological signs including tremors, unstable gait, and abnormal movements. Tests done on the blood and the cerebrospinal fluid showed evidence of rabies virus infection. Her clinical conditions worsened further, with a change in mentation and generalized seizures. However, after a protracted course, the woman made remarkable recovery. The corneal impression taken from this patient was negative for rabies virus. This raises the possibility of the whole clinical picture occurring as a sequelae of the vaccination rather than the rabies infection. The vaccine derived from the brain cells contains foreign antigens and can elicit a violent reaction in susceptible individuals. The body can produce antibodies against the antigen and the antibodies can destroy the patient's own brain and central nervous system. This is called postvaccination encephalomyelitis. This is sometimes difficult to distinguish from rabies. The bizarre neurological feature in this case might point towards a vaccine-related neurological illness rather than actual rabies.

Recovery from Rabies in a Laboratory Worker

The third case of rabies survival was reported in 1977 from New York (Tillotson JR, et al., 1977). A 32-year old laboratory technician was working on developing a technique for mass immunization of wild animals that are susceptible to rabies. The plan was to immunize wild animals on a massive scale, which would greatly reduce their potential to transmit the disease to humans. He was working with a particular rabies strain and was probably infected by aerosols of the virus about 2 weeks prior to the onset of his illness. The team was trying to develop an enteric-coated virus strain. These enteric-coated virus strains were supposed to resist the acid digestion in the wild animals' stomach and impart a certain level of immunity to the virus without infecting them. The experiments involved the use of aerosolized viral particles in a test tube.

He experienced malaise, fatigue, headaches, other generalized body symptoms, and was admitted to the local hospital. A few days after the admission he was unable to talk and slipped into a coma the next day. The blood tests and the tests done on the cerebrospinal fluid were suggestive of rabies. Corneal impression and the skin biopsy did not show any rabies virus. The patient did recover from the coma, albeit slowly. The patient still had residual neurological difficulties with difficulty in speaking and spasticity (increased tone and stiffness of the whole body) 4 months after the illness.

This case points to the danger of aerosolized virus particles. Although rare, it is possible to contract the disease in this form. The aerosolized virus can gain entry into the central nervous system directly through the olfactory nerve endings, rather than the usual peripheral nerves when the individual is bitten on an extremity. Olfactory nerves are very short and pass directly from the nose to the brain. Theoretically, the infection can occur quickly in this situation.

Because of this potential for infection, there are definite guidelines for performing rabies research. Biosafety Level 2 (BSL 2) practices and facilities are recommended for all activities utilizing known or potentially infectious material. BSL 2 practices include limited access, biohazard warning signs, sharps precautions, and a biosafety manual defining waste decontamination or medical surveillance policies. BSL 2 facility immunization is recommended for all individuals prior to working with the rabies virus or with infected animals, or engaging in diagnostic, production, or research activities with the rabies virus.

Cases from Mexico and India

The fourth case occurred in a 9-year-old boy from Mexico (Alvarez L, et al., 1994). The patient was bitten on the face by a rabid dog. He was started on a combination of vaccine and immune globulin treatment as the part of the standard postexposure prophylaxis regimen. But the patient developed fever and difficulty in swallowing 3 weeks after the bite. Subsequently, he developed convulsions and became comatose. The patient was given assistance to breathe with the help of an artificial respirator. Antibody levels in the blood and cerebrospinal fluid were highly suggestive of rabies. The corneal impression smear and the skin biopsy were negative for rabies virus, and the virus was not isolated from the saliva. The boy recovered after several months with severe neurological sequelae including weakness and visual changes.

The fifth case, reported from India, was a 6-year-old girl who made a partial recovery from rabies (Madhusudana SN, et al., 2002). The case was reported from the south Indian city of Bangalore. The girl was bitten on the face by a rabid dog. She was given postexposure prophylaxis. Later, she showed symptoms of rabies and was managed with supportive care only.

Wisconsin 2004: The First Rabies Survivor without Vaccine or Immune Globulin

The sixth and latest case was reported from the United States in 2004 (Willoughby RE, et al., 2005). It is unique in that this was the only case where the patient survived without any form of postexposure prophylaxis. Fifteen-year-old Jeanna Giese picked up a bat while attending a church service in September

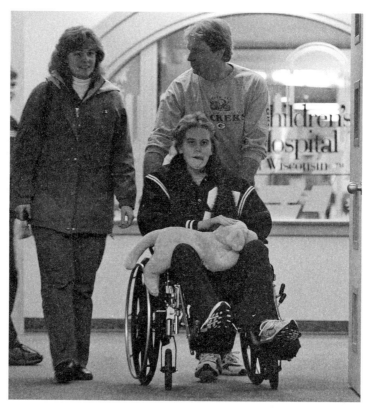

Jenna Giese: The first rabies survivor without vaccine. (AP Photo/Morry Gash)

2004 in Fond du Lac, Wisconsin. She saw the bat falling to the floor, so she picked it up and released it outside the building. The bat was not captured for testing. While holding the bat, she was bitten on the left index finger. There was a 5-mm wound. The wound was cleaned with hydrogen peroxide and no medical attention was sought. Rabies postexposure prophylaxis was not administered.

Thirty-seven days after the bite, she experienced fatigue and paresthesias of the left hand. Two days later, she complained of seeing double. She was unsteady on her feet. She had nausea and vomiting the next day. She progressively developed blurred vision, weakness of the left leg, fever, slurred speech, and tremors. She was transferred to the pediatric infectious disease section of the Medical College of Wisconsin in Milwaukee. The doctors noticed several neurological features such as eye movement abnormalities and tremors of the left arm. The patient was still able to answer questions and comply with simple commands during the examination. Rabies was suspected because of the patient's clinical presentation and the history of bat bite. Samples of the blood, cerebrospinal fluid, and skin biopsy were submitted to the Centers for Disease Control and Prevention (CDC) in Atlanta, Georgia. The patient began to salivate excessively and abnormal swallowing was noted. The patient was connected to a respirator for airway protection. Blood and cerebrospinal fluid tests came back positive for rabies. The rabies virus could not be isolated in the skin biopsy specimen, from saliva, or from cerebrospinal fluid.

At this point, the prognosis seemed poor. The doctors discussed the case with the family and they opted for aggressive treatment. The doctors, after thorough research, formulated a protocol, which later came to be known as the Milwaukee Protocol. The aim was to induce coma and treat the patent with antiviral medications and hope that the body's immunological system would develop its own antibodies that might be able to clear the virus. The doctors administered ketamine and midazolam, two anesthetic agents commonly used in operating rooms to induce a deep coma. Intensive monitoring was done in the intensive care unit to ensure adequate blood supply to the various organs.

Empiric antiviral therapy was given after the induced coma. The drug ribavirin is thought to have some effect against the rabies virus. Ribavirin was administered in the hope that it would penetrate into the brain and destroy the virus. Rabies vaccine or the immune globulin were deliberately not used because the patient was already mounting an immunological response of her own. The doctors feared that a potentiated immunological response might do more harm than good. Amantadine, another antiviral drug, was added to the regimen.

The patient developed several complications during this intensive monitoring in the intensive care unit (ICU). Hemolysis (destruction of the blood inside the body) and acidosis (presence of more acidity in the blood) were noted. The urine output increased because of altered hormonal control. Salivation increased on the eighth day of hospitalization. Paralysis of the intestines was detected. Fever developed and did not respond to the usual treatments. Repeat testing of the cerebrospinal fluid showed increased level of rabies antibody and ketamine was tapered to take the patient slowly out of the induced coma.

On the 12th day, the patient opened her mouth to stimulation. She blinked on instilling eye drops and regained eye movements on the 14th day. On the 19th day she wiggled her toes and squeezed with her hands on command. On the 23rd day the patient sat up in bed, holding her head erect. On day 27, the respirator was discontinued and she was able to breathe without its assistance. On day 30, she cried spontaneously. She was removed from isolation on day 31. She was discharged after 76 days of hospitalization. She continued to improve and after 4 months, she smiled, and was able to talk with some difficulty. She was able to dress herself, eat a normal diet, and attend high school part time. She had generalized abnormal movements known as choreoathetosis.

Eighteen months after the hospitalization, her speech and gait improved significantly. She resumed full-time classes. Learning abilities and memory were normal. The abnormal choreoathetosis disappeared. Twenty-seven months after the hospitalization, she continued to improve, still had some dysarthria (difficulties with speech) and some difficulties in walking (Hu WT, et al., 2007). She took college-level courses in English, physics, and calculus. She scored above average on a national college achievement test and graduated high school with honors in May 2007.

The cause of her remarkable cure is unknown and controversial. The doctors who treated her at the Medical College of Wisconsin claim to have harnessed the body's natural immunity to help clear the virus. They thought the brain pathology in rabies reflected secondary complications possibly from the damage caused by several molecules collectively called excitotoxins. The medications given to their patient (ketamine and midazolam) are known to inhibit two of those well-known excitotoxins. They also praised the aggressive critical care adopted in the case. Complications were promptly detected and addressed. There was previously one case report of a rabies patient maintained alive for 133 days with intensive treatment in the ICU. Ultimately that patient died, but this case pointed the researchers to hypothesize that prolonged monitoring in the ICU is possible. Another reason postulated for this patient's recovery is the possible small amount of virus inoculated into the patient's body because of the small size of the wound. Alternatively, the virus inoculated may be of an attenuated type or a less virulent variety. They could not isolate the virus to confirm or dispute these theories. Dr. Alan Jackson from Queen's University in Ontario, Canada, a prominent rabies researcher, is also doubtful about the effectiveness of the induced coma in the treatment of viral encephalitis such as rabies (Jackson AC, 2005).

The protocol used in the treatment of this patient is known as the Milwaukee Protocol. Dr. Willoughby, who led the team of the doctors treating Jeanna Giese, has initiated a rabies registry at the Wisconsin Medical College website (http://www.mcw.edu/display/router.asp?docid=11655). This site gives the researchers the world over access to the protocol. So far, seven patients have been registered but none have survived the disease, despite using the protocol. Two prominent cases are from the United States.

Indiana 2006: The First U.S. Attempt with the Milwaukee Protocol

A 10-year-old girl complained of pain in the right arm and skin eruptions on September 30, 2006 (CDC, 2006). She developed vomiting and the arm pain increased on October 3. On October 4, a physician was consulted, but

X-rays of the arm and clavicle were normal. Her speech became incoherent and she complained of diminished appetite, sore throat, and neck pain a few days later. She had a fever of 101°F and was irritable and agitated. On October 7, she was admitted to a local community hospital. Her tongue was swollen and symptomatic treatments were given. She had increasing neurological symptoms the next day and was transferred to a tertiary care center. Upon arrival, she was found to have copious salivation and complained of difficulty in swallowing. Because of the concern of choking on saliva and secretions, the patient was connected to a respirator. Empiric treatment with multiple antibiotics was initiated, targeting an infection of the coverings of the brain and the brain itself (meningoencephalitis).

On detailed inquiry, the family members indicated that she had several contacts with healthy appearing household animals such as cats and dogs. A babysitter suggested an animal scratch or bite during June 2006, but this was not substantiated. The patient indicated that she was bitten or scratched by a bat, although she was on a respirator. Samples of serum, saliva, skin biopsies from the nape of the neck, and cerebrospinal fluid samples were sent to the CDC for rabies virus testing. The testing of the blood revealed antibodies against rabies. Rabies virus was identified in the saliva and skin samples.

After the rabies virus infection was confirmed, the patient was started on the Milwaukee Protocol. Aggressive supporting treatment was given in the ICU. Antiexcitatory and antiviral treatment was administered using drugs such as phenobarbital, midazolam, ketamine, amantadine, and ribavirin. Other medications and supplements such as coenzyme Q10, L-arginine, tetrahydrobiopterin, and vitamin C were also administered in hopes of replenishing the good neurotransmitter substances in the brain. The patient was in an induced coma and she developed multiple complications during the hospitalization. The intracranial pressure rose, leading to herniation of the various parts of brain such as the cerebrum and cerebellum. Sedative drugs were withdrawn per the protocol. The patient remained comatose and never regained consciousness. Because of nonimprovement, the life support was withdrawn and the patient died on the 26th day of hospitalization.

The department of public health investigated the antecedents of her illness further. Her mother recollected that in mid-June the girl woke up and told her that a small bird or bat had flown into her bedroom through the open window and bitten her. There was a small mark on the girl's arm and the mother gave her over-the-counter first aid treatment. She checked the girl's room thoroughly. Having found no birds or bats, she assumed that the girl had a nightmare. Two to three days later, one of her siblings found a dead bat with the family cat; however, her mother did not associate this with the previous episode.

The CDC conducted detailed studies on the virus sample obtained from the girl. Detailed genetic testing can give clues to the origins of the virus. This particular strain was found to be a rabies virus variant associated with the silver haired bat, *Lasionycteris noctivagans*. Postexposure prophylaxis was recommended for anyone who came into contact with the patient's saliva from 7 days before the onset of illness to the time of death. A total of 66 individuals were given postexposure prophylaxis. This included seven members of the patient's immediate family, a healthcare worker at the patient's primary care physician's office, nine staff members at the community hospital, an ambulance worker, and 31 individuals from the patient's school and community.

The failure of the protocol in this patient was disappointing. The exact cause is not known. The viral antigen was present in the postmortem samples of the patient's brain. It may be that the patient was unable to mount an antibody response to clear the virus from her system. The premise of the Milwaukee Protocol is that the patient's body system be allowed to mount an antibody response. Moreover, this patient might have had a more virulent strain of rabies because the rabies virus was found in multiple specimens of the patient. That might also indicate a high viral load, leading to a poorer prognosis.

California 2006: The Second Attempt

An 11-year-old boy who was a recent immigrant from the Philippines presented with sore throat, fatigue, and fever on November 15, 2006. He was diagnosed with a case of pharyngitis and the antibiotic amoxicillin was prescribed. The boy developed chest tightness and dysphagia the same evening and was taken to the emergency room (ER). His pulse rate was fast and his blood pressure was elevated. In the ER, the boy exhibited abnormal mouth and lip movements, hallucinations, and agitation. Symptoms such as aerophobia, hydrophobia, and excessive salivation were noted and rabies was suspected. The patient was transferred to a tertiary care pediatric hospital.

The patient was admitted to the ICU. The patient was confused and was unstable. He was administered cardiac support and was connected to a respirator for breathing difficulties. Several samples of the serum, saliva, corneal impression smear, and the cerebrospinal fluid were taken and sent to the CDC for more tests. Rabies virus antigen was detected on the corneal impression smears on November 18. The Milwaukee Protocol was initiated with ketamine, midazolam, ribavirin, amantadine, tetrahydrobiopterin, and coenzyme Q10. The patient developed several complications during this period including fluctuations in heart rate and blood pressure, kidney failure, disturbances in cardiac rhythms, and convulsions. The initial recordings of the brain (electro-encephalogram—EEG) showed a burst suppression pattern indicated by bursts of electrical activity followed by little brain activity. This particular type of activity is seen in the EEG with several conditions such as head trauma, stroke, coma, anoxia, anesthesia, hypothermia, and premature babies. This pattern is related to severe encephalopathy and the prognosis is poor.

On the 21st day of hospitalization the EEG did not show any electrical activity of the brain. On the 24th day severe swelling of the brain developed. The EEG remained flat and on December 13, the patient was disconnected from the respirator. The patient died on the 27th hospital day. Rabies virus antigen was detected on postmortem examination of the brain.

The patient's two siblings reported that a dog bit him approximately 2 years before the onset of the illness while the patient was living in the Philippines. He did not receive any postexposure prophylaxis for rabies at that time. The investigators further studied the genetic makeup of the rabies virus isolated from the boy. The gene sequence was similar to those of rabies viruses seen in dogs in the Philippines. The incubation period of this length (2 years) is unusual in cases of rabies although it is unclear whether the boy had any other recent exposures after the reported one.

This patient did not survive despite the use of the Milwaukee Protocol. Again this virus strain appears to be more virulent; the virus could be isolated from several body sites of the patient. Rabies virus antigen was detected in the brain postmortem, which indicates that the patient failed to eradicate the virus despite an antibody response. The canine virus variant the boy had might also be more virulent than the bat strains of rabies virus.

Dr. Willoughby, the team leader of the doctors who treated the Wisconsin survivor, credits only these two case reports to have closely followed the protocol. He feels that these two patients survived twice as long as the average for rabies patients in the United States. He is also optimistic that we are very close to a second survivor from this fatal disease if more cases follow the protocol. One difficulty in testing the protocol is that an ideal animal model is lacking for this disease. Another drawback is that closely supervised studies of a protocol such as the Milwaukee Protocol are currently almost impossible because there are no animal ICU laboratories where they monitor the infected animals intensely.

Another problem in rabies research is that most of the cases occur in developing countries where resources are scarce and the intensive care treatment that is part of the Milwaukee Protocol is not available to the infected patient. The astronomical cost of the protocol is another stumbling block. Dr. Willoughby reported that he did get several calls inquiring about the protocol, only to be told later that the patient died before the protocol treatment could be arranged.

DECISION ABOUT THE COURSE OF TREATMENT

One of the most important decisions about the treatment of rabies is the course to be taken in an individual patient. Because of the poor prognosis, routine management of rabies should be palliative. Barrier nursing techniques should always be used to limit the contact between the patient and the caregivers and family members. Although transmission of rabies to a health care worker has not been documented to date, the oral secretions from the patient contain significant amounts of the virus. Aggressive therapy as outlined previously may be pursued after detailed discussion with the family members and with the full knowledge that these protocols are experimental in nature and the patient might be left with severe neurological sequelae (Jackson AC, et al., 2003).

Palliative Therapy

Palliative care means any form of medical treatment aimed purely at alleviating the suffering of the patient. Cure of the disease is not the aim. This method is adopted when there is no cure for the disease or when the patient is near the end of life and the patient or the family does not want any aggressive treatment. Palliative therapy is aimed at making the patient comfortable towards the end of life. This is the only modality of treatment available in several parts of the world once the diagnosis of rabies is established. Sedatives, narcotic analgesics, antiepileptic drugs, and neuromuscular blocking drugs are used in various combinations. Phenothiazines, benzodiazepines, or phenobarbital can be used to control the agitation. Carbamazepine can be used to control the seizures. Avoiding stimuli like light, noise, or wind may be humane. Hendekli identifies the following as the cornerstones of good palliative treatment:

1. Excellent access to adequate medicines and equipments.
2. Knowledgeable staff.
3. Barrier nursing techniques.
4. Psychological support for the patient, family, and health care workers.
5. Spiritual/religious support if required (Hendekli, 2005).

Death from rabies can be extremely painful and agonizing if these measures are not used optimally.

6

The Global Burden of Rabies

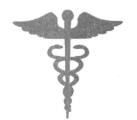

MORE THAN 55,000 PEOPLE DIE EACH YEAR OF RABIES

Although rabies is a vaccine-preventable disease, more than 55,000 people die each year because of rabies. These data are incomplete, suggesting that the death rate may even be higher. Most rabies deaths occur in Asia and Africa, and the majority of the victims are children: 30–50 percent of the reported cases of rabies and deaths occur in children under 15 years of age. The magnitude of this fatality statistic reflects realities on different levels. The developing countries where rabies is endemic are usually poor and unable to afford the costly new generations of vaccines or immune globulin. Several developing countries still use the neural tissue-based vaccine, which is cheap and affordable, but requires several days of return to the hospital for repeated injections, and the compliance rate is low. Moreover, they involve injecting large amounts of the vaccine into the abdominal wall, which can be extremely uncomfortable. The issue of rabies and stray dog control takes a backseat in many countries because of other pressing problems.

EPIDEMIOLOGY OF RABIES ACROSS THE GLOBE

Rabies is also still present in developed countries. In Europe, fewer than five cases are reported in a year. In the United States, one to two cases of rabies occur per year on average. These successes have been achieved by strict prophylactic measures and by means of veterinary rabies control measures in the domestic and wild animal populations. In Europe, the main indigenous animal reservoirs are the dog in eastern European countries and on the borders with the Middle East, the fox in central and eastern Europe, the raccoon dog in northeastern Europe, and the insectivorous bat throughout the entire continent. Rabies virus is transmitted predominantly by dogs in several Asian countries such as Pakistan, China, Indonesia, Thailand, the Philippines, Malaysia, India, and Sri Lanka. Isolation of *Lyssavirus* from bats has been reported in India and Thailand; however, bat rabies is not an endemic problem in these countries. Recently, neutralizing antibodies against rabies virus were detected in six species of bats in the Philippines. This suggests that those bats might have been exposed to rabies virus. The wolf still plays an important role as the vector along with the dog in some regions of Iraq, Iran, Afghanistan, and some countries of the erstwhile Soviet Union. In recent decades the raccoon dog, transported westwards from Siberia for fur and hunting purposes, has become a prolific vector of the disease in western Russia and Poland.

Canine rabies is the predominant type of rabies in Africa. In South Africa, a separate wild cycle of rabies is also found in the yellow mongoose and in the herbivorous kudu antelope. Antelope rabies became established in Namibia in 1977 and claimed the lives of 50,000 antelopes annually until 1983. The disease has spontaneously subsided since then because of unknown reasons, but made a resurgence in 2002 when substantial number of antelopes were affected. Rabies epizootics in Namibia have provided an example of non-bite transmission, with horizontal spread between kudu antelopes. These episodes posed a threat to human health through the game breeding and hunting industries in Namibia.

In Central and South America, canine rabies is the cause of many human deaths and vampire bat rabies is responsible for severe economic losses in cattle. In North America, rabies is enzootic in foxes, skunks, and raccoons. Within these species, compartmentation occurs; that is, the disease is reported in one major host species in certain geographical areas while it is reported much less frequently in the same species in other areas. Rabies in insectivorous bats accounts for 15 percent of all rabies cases in the United States. Spillover of rabies from bats to terrestrial animals occurs more frequently than it was once thought, although there is no suggestion that at present bat rabies viruses cause cycles of disease in terrestrial animals. Despite its relative rarity in industrialized countries, rabies continues to cause significant mortality worldwide with annual deaths estimated at more than 100,000.

RABIES CONTROL IN DOGS

Canine rabies is the most common form of rabies outside of the developed world. Endemic canine rabies contributes to more than 99 percent of all human rabies cases; half of the global human population, especially in the developing world, lives in canine rabies-endemic areas and is considered at risk for contracting rabies. Freely roaming stray dogs compound the problem. They are exposed to wild animals routinely and do not receive rabies vaccine as prophylaxis. The stray dog population proliferates uncontrollably in developing countries. For example, there are believed to be 25 million stray dogs in India without bona fide owners and no proper vaccinations (Sandeep, 2002). The stray dog population is maintained because of the complex sociopolitical environment in the developing countries. The reasons for their prevalence could be:

1. Lack of a proper requirement for pet ownership.
2. Availability of food because of the lack of proper trash disposal.
3. Religious practices or customs.
4. Lack of awareness.
5. Low priority of rabies control in poor areas with other pressing problems.

In developing countries, the awareness of the link between rabies and stray dogs had been acute and several programs in several countries were successful in eliminating the problem of canine rabies. In the 1600s and 1700s, dogs in Europe and North America were extensively used for hunting in packs. During this sort of hunting, widespread exposure to rabies occurred in several animals at the same time. Wild foxes played an important part in transmitting the infection in this way. Killing the whole pack of foxes exposed to rabies was a last resort to control the spread of infection. Strict reporting and elimination of diseased dogs existed in several European cities during these periods, which also helped in preventing the spread of the disease. Nineteenth-century Europe perfected these techniques with isolation, leashing, or even muzzling of animals suspected of rabies. The Scandinavian countries became canine rabies-free towards the end of the 19th century. Countries of western and central Europe followed suit in the early 20th century, although there were a few cases that surfaced after the two world wars.

Vaccination of stray dogs was a controversial technique earlier in the last century. Most control programs relied on shooting or poisoning of the stray dog population. The campaigns in Japan, Hungary, and Malaysia proved that mass vaccination of dogs can prevent and eliminate canine rabies. Several countries resorted to eliminating dogs in order to be free from rabies. Animal rights groups protested against this and lobbied for a more humane treatment of dogs to control rabies. A combination of dog control and vaccination adapted to the national and local conditions was advised as the optimal solution. In 2008, officials in the north Indian city of Srinagar in Kashmir planned to kill all 100,000 stray dogs roaming the city. They claimed that these free-roaming animals had become a menace for the people, making urban life unbearable. The poison intended was strychnine, a neurotoxin that will paralyze and cripple an animal in a short time. Animal advocates stated that the sight of the deaths of these animals in full public view would be unbearable and inhumane. Municipal authorities later halted the program after the animal rights campaigners threatened court action on the grounds of cruelty. In 2007, Egypt also decided to control the burgeoning population of stray dogs in Cairo's twin city of Giza by shooting and poisoning the animals, because it was cheaper than sterilization. The authorities estimated that sterilizing the dogs would cost $10.49 million a year whereas shooting them only required $80,678 (The Australian, 2007).

Dog Killing Is Not the Answer

In Mouding County in Yunnan province in southwestern China, 50,000 dogs were killed in a government-ordered crackdown after three people died of rabies. This 5-day slaughter spared only military guard dogs and police canine units. Dogs being walked were seized from their owners and beaten to death on the spot. The "killing teams" entered villages at night, creating noise to get dogs barking, and then beat the animals to death. These mass killings were widely condemned. In 2007, Ethiopian authorities in Addis Ababa also planned to kill tens of thousands of stray dogs in the Ethiopian capital using strychnine-laced meat, saying that they wanted to eradicate rabies before a local festival. The killing of stray animals is fundamentally flawed in that the extermination attempts are never complete, and the remaining dogs or other dogs from the neighboring areas migrate to fill in the ecological niche. The usual success rate of these elimination campaigns is only 4–6 percent annually. In one of the extreme efforts, 24 percent of the dog population was removed in Guayaquil, Ecuador, yet no significant effect on the stray dog population and rabies incidence were noted (Jackson and Wunner, 2002, 434). An annual turnover of 30–40 percent of dog population is considered normal in countries where stray dogs are common. The World Health Organization (WHO) advocates Animal Birth Control (ABC) as a humane method of reducing dog populations and rabies control. In the ABC program, street dogs are captured, sterilized, vaccinated against rabies, and released back to the area from where they were captured. The ABC strategy is already in effect in many countries of the world including Sri Lanka, Indonesia, India, United Arab Emirates, Egypt, Brazil, Greece, Kenya, and Turkey (WHO, 2005). In India, which has the highest instances of rabies and dog-bite cases in south Asia, ABC has been the official government policy for some time now, including several major cities.

The ABC program is possible with aggressive catching and vaccination of stray dogs. In Lima, Peru, with a high incidence of rabies, 273,000 dogs and 54,000 cats were vaccinated in 1 month. Several of these animals were strays. This campaign covered 65 percent of the estimated dog population in addition to the 12.7 percent already vaccinated. Total vaccination coverage for the whole population was 77.7 percent. Rabies disappeared for several years. A Philippines campaign led by WHO in 1994 also documented the feasibility of vaccinating large numbers of dogs. A combination of public awareness programs and interdisciplinary collaboration is also important in eliminating canine rabies from developing countries. South America has success stories in Uruguay and Chile. Uruguay became rabies-free in 1983 and Chile succeeded in eliminating dog rabies. During the past 20 years, the number of human and canine rabies cases in South America has declined by nearly 90 percent.

Today, with large areas of Europe gaining rabies-free status, vaccination of pets nevertheless remains an important part of prevention. Travel with pets from countries with endemic wildlife and dog-mediated rabies is a risk for public health and can result in re-infection of the previously rabies-free areas. Therefore, strict laws and regulations have been implemented to control the movement of pet animals (e.g., dogs, cats, and ferrets). They have to be vaccinated before travel and a sufficient immune response has to be achieved.

CONTROL OF FOX RABIES IN EUROPE

Rabies in Europe is predominantly sylvatic rabies (a rabies cycle that affects only wild animals), with wildlife species accounting for approximately 80 percent of all rabies cases. Red foxes (*Vulpes vulpes*) are responsible for about 80 percent of such cases. Conventional methods, such as intensive culling or trapping of foxes, were previously used to disrupt their natural route of infection by reducing their population density. These methods were generally incapable of reducing and maintaining the fox population below a certain level. The oral vaccination of foxes provided an exciting new opportunity to control the incidence of rabies in foxes. This technique was developed 25 years ago. The first field trials were conducted in Switzerland in 1978.

In the face of advancing fox rabies, a Swiss team lead by Steck and colleagues used a modified live rabies virus vaccine strain called SAD-Berne to prevent the spread of rabies into the country. Initial trials were conducted on a river island near the town of Solothurn. The aim was to conduct a field trial after numerous trials of SAD virus pathogenicity were carried out under laboratory conditions. After intense baiting all over the island, 760 rodents were trapped and virologically examined. No rabies or rabies-like viruses were detected.

Following this trial, in October 1978, relying on the barrier effect of surrounding alpine chains, an attempt was made to stop the progression of an advancing rabies epizootic by laying vaccine baits in a strip 60 km wide and 8 km long, blocking the entrance of the Rhone valley (Wandeler, et al., 1988). The vaccine baits consisted of chicken heads with a plastic and aluminum capsule filled with 1.8 mL of SAD virus solution clipped under the skin. Laying of the vaccine baits was repeated during spring and autumn of the following years. Tetracycline examinations in the bones of the foxes killed in the area confirmed that 60 percent of the population had eaten the baits. Switzerland remained free of fox rabies. For the first time, it was possible to prevent the entry of rabies into an isolated area by the oral vaccination of foxes, and to eliminate an invading disease in wildlife only by vaccination.

Germany followed this by conducting similar trials in 1983. Since then, this method has been proven as the only effective way to eliminate rabies in foxes and other terrestrial reservoir species. If rabies is eliminated in foxes, it also disappears in domestic animals. The results of these trials are remarkable. The annual number of rabies cases in Europe dropped from 21,000 in the year 1990 to 5,400 in 2004. Most parts of western and central Europe successfully controlled and eradicated rabies. Several countries such as Finland and The Netherlands (1991), Italy (1997), Switzerland (1998), France (2000), Belgium, Luxembourg (2001), and the Czech Republic (2004) have been declared as officially free of terrestrial rabies. For oral vaccination of foxes, modified live virus rabies vaccines in the form of either attenuated live rabies viruses or recombinant viruses are used. A vaccine-filled sachet is enveloped by a bait casing typically consisting of fishmeal, fat, and paraffin.

ORAL RABIES VACCINATION IN NORTH AMERICA (UNITED STATES AND CANADA)

Oral rabies vaccination (ORV) has been under field investigation in Canada since 1985 and in the United States since 1990. Currently, there are 15 states distributing oral vaccines for raccoons in the United States. Texas distributes baits for the gray fox and coyote as well. Raboral V-RG® is the only effective oral vaccine licensed for use in free-ranging raccoons, gray foxes, and coyotes in the United States. Merial, Ltd., in Iselin, New Jersey, manufactures Raboral V-RG. Nearly 48 million doses of Raboral V-RG have been distributed in the United States and Canada, and 63 million doses have been dispersed worldwide.

V-RG is a recombinant vaccine made from a living pox virus vector, vaccinia (V), which carries the rabies antigen in the form of rabies glycoprotein (RG). The RG is the protective sheath that surrounds the rabies virus. This protein elicits an immune response when swallowed by raccoons, gray foxes, or coyotes. When a raccoon bites oral rabies vaccine bait, the V virus, which is part of the vaccine bait, enters the raccoon's cells. The cells then produce a part of the rabies virus called rabies virus glycoprotein. This stimulates the raccoon's immune system to begin producing disease-fighting antibodies against the rabies virus. The vaccine cannot cause rabies by itself because it contains only the non-infective surface proteins of the rabies virus, not the whole viral nuclear material that is necessary for the virus to replicate and cause an infection. This is generally safe, but pregnant and immunodeficient individuals should avoid touching the vaccine because they might develop a localized pox-like infection. This is characterized by formation of small blebs in the skin. These vaccines are not useful to immunize domestic animals; they are effective only in wild animals (North Carolina Public Health, 2008).

The outer bait matrix is made from fishmeal (for raccoons and coyotes) or dog food (for gray foxes) combined with a polymer that acts as a binding agent. The vaccine packet, or sachet, resembles a small ketchup or mustard package from a fast food restaurant and contains about 1.5 mL of vaccine. The sachet is inside the bait matrix and waxed into place so it does not fall out during aerial delivery. A label printed in black on baits available in the United States reads: "RABIES VACCINE / LIVE VACCINIA VECTOR / DO NOT DISTURB / 1-877-722-6725." As the raccoon, gray fox, or coyote eats through the outer bait matrix, the inner sachet gets punctured, allowing the vaccine to enter the animal's mouth and coat the lymphatic tissue in the throat. There is an immune response to the rabies antigen that creates antibodies to fight off the disease. After 2–3 weeks the animal develops rabies antibodies and is immune to the disease, thus stopping the spread of rabies.

Vaccine baits need to be deposited throughout all potential fox habitats (i.e., almost everywhere). Baits are distributed by aircraft or helicopter in rural areas and forests and by hand in urban and suburban areas. Airplanes fly in straight lines or "transects" at about 500 feet above ground while distributing baits. The bait distribution machine is controlled from the airplane and is turned off when crossing a road or house to avoid human contact with the bait. Baiting by hand is done in busy urban and suburban areas (city parks, cemeteries, industrial areas, private properties, etc.) to decrease human contact with baits. In 2003, more than 10 million baits were distributed in the United States and Canada.

The National Oral Rabies Vaccination (ORV) Program has the goal of limiting the westward expansion of raccoon rabies from the east coast of the United States. This is being accomplished through the establishment of a "vaccine barrier" that will run from eastern Ohio (beginning at the border with Lake Erie) down the Appalachian ridge to Mobile County, Alabama, ending at the Gulf of Mexico.

MENACE TO THE TRAVELER

The large numbers of stray dogs pose a danger to travelers to developing countries. A few recent cases can attest to this risk. Travelers engaged in extensive unprotected outdoor activities such as bicycling, camping, hiking, or engaging in certain occupational activities might be at higher risk even if their trip is brief. Children are considered at higher risk because of their tendencies to play with animals and to not report bites. Casual exposure to cave air is not a concern, but cavers should be warned not to handle any bats.

ENGLAND 2001: TRAVELER RETURNING FROM PHILIPPINES

A British patient presented to a London hospital with aching and numbness at the site of a dog bite sustained during a recent trip to the Philippines. He was bitten during a fight between two dogs in the Philippines 6 weeks earlier. He did not seek medical treatment following the bite. Both dogs involved in the fight had died, alerting the patient to the possibility that he might be at risk of rabies. He developed difficulty in swallowing and spasms of the face and throat. He was diagnosed to have rabies and succumbed to his illness. Health care staff and other close contacts of the patient were offered rabies postexposure prophylaxis as a precaution.

Rabies is found in animals in many countries, but the United Kingdom (UK) has been entirely free of rabies since the early 1920s. The last human case of rabies acquired in the UK was in 1902. Between 1976, when rabies became a statutorily notifiable disease, and 2000, nine deaths from rabies were reported. None of the cases were acquired in the UK. All of these rabies infections were acquired from abroad (Health Protection Agency, 2005).

Austria 2004: Vacationing in Morocco

Two Austrian tourists (a 23-year-old man and a 21-year-old woman) were visiting Agadir, Morocco, in May 2004 (Krause, et al., 2005). In July, they were playing with stray puppies at the beach. One aggressive puppy bit the woman on the hand. While trying to help her, the man was also bitten on the right hand and the leg. The wounds healed naturally and no medical attention was sought. Three days later, the dog died, and was buried by the tourists.

Four weeks later, the man fell ill with fever, malaise, headache, dry mouth and difficulty in swallowing. He was admitted to a hospital in Ceuta, which is a Spanish enclave in mainland Morocco, just opposite to Gibraltar. He was agitated and salivated profusely, demonstrating hydrophobia and aerophobia. His blood pressure became unsteady and his respiratory rate increased. The patient was admitted to the intensive care unit and was connected to a respirator because of breathing difficulties. Supportive treatment with medications to increase the blood pressure was given. Rabies was suspected because of the history of the dog bite and the subsequent death of the dog. His girlfriend remained healthy. Both were administered the rabies vaccination and immune globulin. The patient also developed pneumonia as a complication and was given antibiotics. Three days later, he was transferred by air ambulance to the intensive care unit at the Medical University of Graz, Austria. Intensive treatment including antibiotics for the pneumonia was continued. Midazolam and ketamine were also given as per the recommendations at that time. Skin biopsy specimens from the neck and pharyngeal swabs were positive for rabies virus. The virus was very similar to the strain prevalent in Morocco. The blood tests were also positive for rabies.

The patient worsened in the intensive care unit. The pupils of the patient were fixed and not showing any reaction to a light source exposure. Two electroencephalograms showed no brain activity on day 20. Life support was discontinued and the patient died 27 days after the onset of rabies symptoms. The female partner of the patient was also admitted to the hospital because the same rabid dog also bit her. She remained normal. Rabies vaccination, which had been started in Ceuta, was continued. She was discharged from the hospital in healthy condition.

Interestingly, around this time French authorities reported that a rabid dog had been illegally imported into France from Agadir, Morocco, in July 2004. The Austrian patient also acquired rabies from the same city in July. WHO reported in September 2004 that the rabid dog in France was aggressive and had bitten several people. French authorities contacted several persons and offered counseling and postexposure prophylaxis. No cases of rabies associated with this particular dog were reported. This story underlines the importance of travel-associated rabies and the need for awareness of tourists to rabies-endemic areas about the potential of disease transmission from animals, such as stray dogs and wild animals. Austrian researchers felt that the general public in Austria does not consider rabies to be a serious problem, and that the recommendations for vaccination of travelers to rabies-endemic countries are sometimes ignored.

Germany 2004: Rabies Cases after Visiting India

There were two cases of imported rabies in Germany in 2004 (Health Protection Agency, 2006). A 51-year-old man from Bavaria contracted rabies 6 weeks after returning from a 5-month stay in India. He had contacts with stray dogs and had been bitten once by a monkey while in India. No treatment was sought. The man developed hydrophobia, pharyngeal spasms, and respiratory failure after coming back to Germany. He died 20 days after the onset of symptoms. Investigators could not ascertain whether the exposure was due to the monkey bite or through contact with the saliva of infected dogs.

The other case was that of a German woman who died of rabies after spending 4 weeks in India in late December 2004. The patient was originally admitted to the psychiatric ward because of mental status changes and subsequently her condition worsened and the patient died of cardiorespiratory arrest. The organs of this patient were transplanted into six recipients (two corneal transplants, one liver transplant, one pancreas transplant, and two kidney transplant recipients). On February 16, 2005, the Deutsche Stiftung Organtransplantation (German Foundation for Organ Transplantation) reported possible rabies in three of six patients who received organs from the donor. Two of the three patients who received lung and kidney transplants died after developing progressive neurological symptoms. The third patient who received kidney/pancreas transplants remained in critical condition. All three patients tested positive for rabies virus. The remaining three organ recipients (two corneal, one liver) have not yet shown any signs of rabies. Tests on samples from these three have so far been negative for rabies. The two recipients of the corneas underwent excision and removal of the grafts and received postexposure prophylaxis. The recipient of the liver had been vaccinated prophylactically several years before the transplant and he also received postexposure prophylaxis following the surgery.

As a precaution, all contacts of the infected donor and the infected patients in Germany received rabies immune globulin and started a course of rabies vaccination. A warning was posted on the European Early Warning and Response System on February 18. Rabies was confirmed in the donor patient postmortem. There were no clinical indications to suggest that the donor was infected with rabies prior to her death from cardiac arrest at the hospital. The donor is thought to have acquired the infection during a trip to India in October 2004. The difficulty of diagnosing rabies in unfamiliar circumstances and the absence of a witnessed account of exposure to rabies led to the acceptance of the young German woman as an organ donor. The international agencies have further tightened the regulations and requirements of organ transplantation to prevent such calamities in future.

England 2004: 2-Week Vacation in India

A 39-year-old woman from Bury, Greater Manchester, was bitten by a dog in Goa and became unwell after her return to the UK (Solomon, et al., 2005). Initially, the patient was admitted to her local general hospital under the orthopedic surgeons, complaining of lower back pain radiating to the left leg of 4 days' duration. The pain was shooting in nature. She had two emergency room visits for the same. Subsequently, she became unable to walk. She also complained of a headache and had vomited once. She had vacationed for 2 weeks in Goa, India about 3.5 months before admission. During that time, a dog bit her. She was walking in the street when a puppy on a lead nipped her on the left leg. The resulting slight graze was wiped with a tissue, and she did not seek any medical help. Her family reported that she was not aware of the risk of rabies and had not received any pre-exposure or postexposure vaccination.

Physical examination showed an extremely painful left leg with no reflexes, as well as weakness and sensory loss. Morphine was given for the excruciating pain. The white cell count in the blood was elevated. A computed tomographic scan of the spine looking for a prolapsed vertebral disk was normal. She developed a sore throat and had difficulty swallowing during the course of next several days. She also developed swelling of the left eyelid and hearing loss in both ears. The patient was referred to the medical team on day 8. She was lethargic and had flaccid weakness of both arms and legs. A provisional diagnosis of Guillain–Barré syndrome was considered and treatment with intravenous immunoglobulin was given.

A lumbar puncture found clear cerebrospinal fluid with a minimally elevated white cell count of 11 cells/μL (9 lymphocytes, 2 polymorphnuclear cells). By day 11, the patient was worsening with increasing drowsiness. She was connected to a respirator. On day 13, she had absent oculocephalic reflexes, unreactive pupils, and a diagnosis of Bickerstaff's encephalitis was considered. This is a form of Guillain–Barré syndrome, which also has some inflammation of the brainstem. A computed tomographic scan of the brain was normal.

On the 15th day of admission, the infectious diseases unit and specialist neurology center were contacted for advice. Because of the history of ascending paralysis and history of a dog bite in India, rabies was considered a possibility and tests were ordered. Tests on saliva were reported as positive for rabies. She was diagnosed with rabies and had treatment at the Walton Centre for Neurology in Liverpool. A detailed study of the virus genome proved that it was a strain common in India. A skin biopsy from the nape of the neck also tested positive for the rabies virus. Once the diagnosis was confirmed, the respirator and other supports were withdrawn at the family's request, and the patient died on the 18th day of hospitalization. She never exhibited hydrophobia, aerophobia (fear of air), hypersalivation, or spasms. With the family's permission, brain tissue was obtained after death by needle biopsies through the foramen magnum and supraorbital routes; the presence of rabies virus was confirmed on these specimens. Rising antirabies antibody titers were found in the serum, as measured by the fluorescent virus neutralization assay.

Germany 2007: Dog Bite in Morocco

A 55-year-old man presented to a local hospital in Germany with fever, nausea, altered feelings of the left hand, headache, and difficulty in swallowing on April 17, 2007 (Schmiedel, et al., 2007). He had traveled to Morocco 6 weeks before and his pet dog had been involved in a fight with a stray dog in Morocco. The stray dog also bit the patient's left hand while he was trying to separate the fighting dogs. Medical consultation was sought immediately after the injury, but no rabies vaccination was initiated. Four weeks later, on return to Germany, the patient's dog developed inability to stand up and was euthanized.

Rabies was suspected in the man because of the clinical presentation and the history of the dog bite in Morocco. The patient was referred to University Medical Centre of Hamburg, Germany, on April 18, 2007. On admission in Hamburg, the tests for rabies virus in two different saliva samples and one corneal impression were positive. The genotyping of the virus showed significant matching with the rabies virus type prevalent in Morocco. The patient had received active and passive postexposure vaccination in the local hospital on April 17, 2007. Deep sedation with ketamine and midazolam was initiated on April 19, 2007. Amantadine was also given. Despite all of the efforts, the patient succumbed to the disease because of multiorgan failure on May 14th.

Netherlands 2007: 2-Week Holiday in Kenya

A 34-year-old female doctor was admitted to the Academic Medical Center of the University of Amsterdam in the Netherlands on November 19, 2007 with difficulty in speaking, increased sensation of both cheeks, and unsteady gait (van Thiel, et al., 2008). Her symptoms started 1 day prior to admission. She also had nausea, dizziness, and general malaise for a few days prior to the admission. On October 24, 2007, at the start of a 2-week holiday trip through Kenya, a small bat had flown against her face. She tried to hit away the animal, but it made two bleeding scratches on the right side of her nose. This incident happened at a camping site between Nairobi and Mombasa, at dusk, while she was brushing her teeth. She washed the wound with soap and cleaned with alcohol. The local Kenyan medical personnel were unaware of bat rabies in the locale and did not advise any further action. The woman and her husband continued their vacation.

The possibility of rabies was considered on admission, and postexposure treatment was initiated. Diagnosis of infection with *Lyssavirus*, genotype 4–Duvenhage virus (DUVV) was confirmed in a nuchal biopsy taken on the second day of admission. This is a bat-type rabies virus prevalent in Africa. The patient's neurological status deteriorated rapidly. After consultation with the family, Milwaukee rabies treatment protocol was initiated with induction of deep coma. Despite extreme efforts, the patient died on December 8, 2007, 23 days after the onset of illness. Altogether, 25 close family contacts and 30 attending hospital employees were given active postexposure prophylaxis.

As exemplified from the previous examples, there are risks associated with travel to rabies-endemic countries. Travelers should avoid all unnecessary contact with any animals. Even pet animals from developed countries might not be regularly vaccinated. If bitten or scratched by a warm-blooded animal, travelers should wash the wound with plenty of soap and water and seek medical attention immediately, even if they were previously vaccinated. If they do not seek medical treatment while abroad, they should seek it when they return to their home country, even if it is some time after the event. Promptly administered, postexposure prophylaxis is extremely effective in preventing rabies. Individuals who have not received any rabies vaccine prior to a potential exposure should receive a postexposure prophylaxis consisting of a dose of vaccine as soon as possible after the bite followed by four further doses 3, 7, 14, and 30 days later. If the person has been vaccinated previously, fewer doses of vaccine are advised. Human rabies immune globulin may also be given if the exposure is considered to be high risk.

Travel agents need to stress the importance of obtaining travel health advice well before holidays or trips overseas. All risks associated with travel should be disclosed to the prospective traveler. Rabies is only one of the many challenges faced by a traveler in a foreign land. Rabies vaccine is not routinely advised for all travelers in the UK. Pre-exposure immunization for rabies is recommended for those living in or traveling for more than 1 month to rabies-enzootic areas, unless there is reliable access to prompt, safe medical services; those traveling for less than 1 month in rabies-enzootic areas but who may be exposed to rabies because of their travel activities; and those who have limited access to postexposure medical services in the country in which they travel.

Advice for Travelers to Rabies-Endemic Countries

The UK authorities recommend that travelers to rabies-endemic countries consult their primary care physicians and explain the details of their travel plans. Several other resources such as travel health clinics, the current edition of *Immunization against Infectious Disease*, and consultants in communicable disease control are also available. When traveling, the advice is to stay away from all animals, particularly dogs, cats, and bats. Wild animals that normally avoid humans can appear tame when infected with the rabies virus. This should be remembered before attempting to pet or catch such animals. If a bite, scratch, or other close contact with an animal (including bats) occurs, wash the wound immediately with plenty of soap and water. Note the identity of the animal and its owner when known. The animal may be vaccinated and should be observed to see whether it develops rabies and dies. Vaccination of the traveler should be started until the situation can be fully assessed. Travelers are advised to obtain the advice of a qualified local doctor immediately. It may be necessary to travel to a nearby major city to obtain expert advice. They may recommend postexposure vaccination. The travelers are advised to bring records of all such treatments back to the UK. The names and dates of any vaccine or immune globulin given should be noted correctly. The travelers should immediately consult their general practitioner upon return so doctors can make sure that the correct vaccines were administered and complete the course, if necessary. Travelers are reminded that postexposure prophylaxis is extremely effective in preventing rabies, even when the immunization has had to be delayed for a few days. Vaccine and immune globulin for pre- and postexposure prophylaxis is available from the Public Health Laboratory Services in the UK, free of charge, if vaccination is recommended per the current guidelines.

The UK has been rabies-free for several years and there has been strict enforcement of the movements of animals and pets into the country. The disease in animals is most likely to be introduced either through a smuggled pet or the failure to detect and detain a noncompliant "Pet Travel Scheme" animal. European Bat Lyssavirus (EBLV), which has been found in bats in UK, is not the same rabies strain as that carried by animals like cats, dogs, and foxes. EBLV very rarely crosses the species barrier from bats to other animals or humans. There have been no recorded cases of rabies in UK wildlife or pet animals since EBLV was first identified in a bat in the UK in 1996. The UK is currently free of classical rabies, but a type of rabies virus called the European Bat Lyssavirus type 2 (EBLV-2) is present in UK's Daubenton's bats. There have been four cases of EBLV-2 in Daubenton's bats (*Myotis daubentonii*) in the UK between 1996 and 2004 and approximately 4 percent of healthy Daubenton's bats are seropositive. EBLVs have been responsible for four human deaths in Europe, including the death of a bat conservationist in Scotland in November 2002 (BBC News, 2002).

Pet Imports to UK

The European Union (EU) has restrictions in place relating to the noncommercial movement of pet animals into and around the EU. The UK has additional restrictions in place to prevent the introduction of rabies into the country (Department for Environment, Food, and Rural Affairs, 2008). These include the "Pet Travel Scheme" (PETS) as well as specified quarantine measures for susceptible imported animals. The Department of Environment, Food, and Rural Affairs (DEFRA) has published detailed guidelines for bringing pets into the UK. Individuals have to bring a pet dog, cat, or ferret into (or back into) the UK through PETS without putting it into quarantine. It also explains the requirements for bringing many other types of pet animals into the UK. This site also tells about quarantine in the UK for animals that do not qualify for PETS. These almost draconian measures help to keep the UK rabies free.

PETS

PETS is the system that allows pet dogs, cats, and ferrets from certain countries to enter the UK without quarantine, as long as they meet the rules. This scheme also covers pets such as dogs, cats, and ferrets taken to other EU countries and returned to the UK. This also applies for returning from certain non-EU countries, without the need for quarantine. The rules are designed to keep the UK free from rabies and certain other diseases. PETS was introduced for dogs and cats traveling from certain European countries in 2000. The scheme was extended to Cyprus, Malta, and certain long-haul countries in 2001. Bahrain, mainland United States, and Canada joined in 2002. The EU regulation on the movements of pet animals extended the scheme to include ferrets and increased the number of qualifying (listed) countries.

The European regulation, which sets the rules for dogs, cats, and ferrets to travel between European Community countries, and into the community from other countries, also covers the movement of other pet animals: Movement between EU countries or into the EU from Andorra, Iceland, Liechtenstein, Monaco, Norway, San Marino, Switzerland, and the Vatican are not subject to any requirement with regard to rabies. Currently there are no requirements for these animals when entering the UK from any of these countries. When imported into the UK from any non-EU country, other than those listed in the previous paragraph, pets must be licensed into quarantine for 6 months. Importation of prairie dogs originating in or traveling from the United States into the EU is prohibited. It also prohibits the import of certain rodents and squirrels originating in or traveling from certain countries of the sub-Saharan region of Africa.

The EU regulation on the movement of pet animals also covers birds (except certain poultry), ornamental tropical fish, invertebrates (except bees and crustaceans), amphibians, and reptiles. To bring these animals into the UK, they must meet either national import rules or the general rules for trade in the animal species.

It is against the law in Great Britain to possess certain types of animals, and meeting the requirements of PETS does not change that. Domestic dogs and cats are not covered by the Dangerous Wild Animals Act but certain hybrid dogs and cats (bred through crossing domestic animals with wild species) may be subject to its provisions. The Dangerous Dogs Act of 1991 prohibits four types of dogs: pit bull terrier, Japanese tosa, dogo argentino, and fila brasileiro. A host of other animals requires license if kept as private animals. The Dangerous Wild Animals Act 1976, modified in 2007, provides detailed guidelines.

The UK does not permit the import of dogs, cats, and ferrets that have not been vaccinated against rabies. Once they have reached the minimum age for vaccination (as stated on the vaccine manufacturer's data sheet) they must be vaccinated against rabies before being taken to the UK. A detailed list of the EU and non-EU countries from where the importation is permitted per PETS is available at http://www.defra.gov.uk/animalh/quarantine/pets/territory.htm. Dogs, cats, and ferrets must not have been outside any of these countries in the 6 calendar months before entering the UK. Before traveling, people must ensure that pet cats and dogs (including assistance dogs) and ferrets meet all of the rules of PETS. Dogs, cats, and ferrets entering the UK under PETS may do so only through certain sea, air, and rail routes.

Rabies Quarantine

Dogs, cats, and ferrets entering the UK from nonqualifying (unlisted) countries must spend 6 months in quarantine upon arrival. The detailed quarantine process begins with the reservation of quarantine accommodation for the pet at the traveler's choice. Usually these premises will take care of arrangements, such as submitting an application form for an import license to Animal Health (formerly the State Veterinary Service), arranging to collect the pet at the port or airport of landing, clearance through customs, and safe custody to the quarantine premises. The list of authorized quarantine premises and authorized carrying agents is available on the DEFRA website. Animals going into quarantine may only be landed at certain ports/airports. The maximum number of all types of pet animals (not only rabbits and rodents) each person may bring into the EU from most non-EU listed countries is five. This rule does not apply to animals brought from Andorra, Iceland, Liechtenstein, Monaco, Norway, San Marino, Switzerland, or the Vatican.

The quarantine website provides information about rabies quarantine in the UK for cats, dogs, and other rabies-susceptible animals that do not qualify for entry into the UK under PETS and are required by law to spend 6 months in quarantine (Department for Environment, Food, and Rural Affairs, 2008).

CONFIRMED RABIES CASE IN DOG IN FRANCE

Authorities in both the UK and France announced a confirmed case of rabies in a dog (young mixed-breed female) in Paris, France, in 2007. The dog had direct contact with another dog (black cross Labrador) belonging to the same family, which died in early January. The mixed-breed dog died on February 19, setting off an investigation. The Labrador had been in contact with a third dog (a mixed-breed border collie) that entered France from Morocco in late October 2006 and then died in Gers, southwest France, in mid-November. Both the Labrador and the Moroccan dog showed symptoms compatible with rabies. The French authorities investigated movements of all three dogs and have identified four potential risk areas in different parts of France where people may have been exposed to rabies. The risk to humans was considered low. However, health authorities in both countries advised anyone who might have sustained a dog bite while traveling or staying in the regions of France during those periods to seek prompt medical advice. This sort of collaboration shows the seriousness and effectiveness of international cooperation and coordinated efforts to prevent the spread of rabies.

ANIMAL IMPORT REGULATIONS IN THE UNITED STATES

The Centers for Disease Control and Prevention (CDC) regulations govern the importation of dogs, cats, turtles, monkeys, other animals, and animal products capable of causing human disease into the United States. Requirements for the importation of the most common pets are described below. Pets taken out of the United States are subject upon return to the same regulations as those entering for the first time.

The CDC does not require general certificates of health for pets entering the United States. However, health certificates may be required for entry into some states or may be required by the airlines. Importation of certain animals as pets is prohibited. Special license is required to import animals such as monkeys, other primates, and bats. Bats require a quarantine of 6 months after importation.

Pet dogs are subject to inspection at ports of entry and may be denied entry into the United States if they have evidence of an infectious disease that can be transmitted to humans. If a dog appears ill, further examination by a licensed veterinarian might be required at the port of entry. Dogs must have a certificate showing that they have been vaccinated against rabies at least 30 days prior to entry into the United States. Puppies less than 3 months of age that are too young to be vaccinated must be kept in confinement until they are old enough to be vaccinated and then confined for at least 30 days after the date of vaccination. Unvaccinated dogs must be vaccinated within 4 days of arrival at their final U.S. destination and within 10 days of entry into the United States and must be kept in confinement for at least 30 days after the date of vaccination. Unvaccinated dogs may be imported without a requirement for proof of rabies vaccination if they have been located for a minimum of 6 months or more in countries that are free of rabies. A current list of rabies-free countries is given in Table 6.1.

Table 6.1.
Countries and Political Units Reporting No Indigenous Cases of Rabies during 2005 (adopted from CDC, 2008a).

Region	Countries
Africa	Cape Verde, Libya, Mauritius, Réunion, São Tome and Principe, and Seychelles
Americas	North: Bermuda, St. Pierre, and Miquelon
	Caribbean: Antigua and Barbuda, Aruba, Bahamas, Barbados, Cayman Islands, Dominica, Guadeloupe, Jamaica, Martinique, Montserrat, Netherlands Antilles, Saint Kitts (Saint Christopher) and Nevis, Saint Lucia, Saint Martin, Saint Vincent and Grenadines, Turks and Caicos, and Virgin Islands (UK and U.S.)
	South: Uruguay
Asia	Hong Kong, Japan, Kuwait, Lebanon, Malaysia (Sabah), Qatar, Singapore, United Arab Emirates
Europe	Austria, Belgium, Cyprus, Czech Republic[1], Denmark[1], Finland, France[1], Gibraltar, Greece, Iceland, Ireland, Isle of Man, Italy, Luxemburg, Netherlands[1], Norway, Portugal, Spain[1] (except Ceuta/ Melilla), Sweden, Switzerland, and United Kingdom[1]
Oceania	Australia[1], Northern Mariana Islands, Cook Islands, Fiji, French Polynesia, Guam, Hawaii, Kiribati, Micronesia, New Caledonia, New Zealand, Palau, Papua New Guinea, Samoa, and Vanuatu

[1]Bat lyssaviruses are known to exist in these areas that are reportedly free of rabies in other animals.

CDC does not require a general certificate of health for entry of pet cats into the United States, although some airlines or states may require them. Pet cats are subject to inspection at ports of entry and may be denied entry into the United States if they have evidence of an infectious disease that can be transmitted to humans. If a cat appears to be ill, further examination by a licensed veterinarian at the owner's expense might be required at the port of entry. Cats are not required to have proof of rabies vaccination for importation into the United States. However, some states require vaccination of cats for rabies, so it may be worthwhile to check with the state or local authorities about the relevant rules before importing a pet cat.

These regulations are designed to prevent the spread of various infectious agents including rabies. The ultimate success of such regulations depends not only on the meticulous application of the relevant laws, but also eradication of rabies from the largest reservoirs, mostly in developing countries.

RABNET

WHO has been collecting rabies data electronically on a yearly basis through Rabnet, an interactive information system able to generate interactive maps and graphs using human and animal rabies data. Two years ago, Rabnet version 2 was launched. Online data entry and updating could be done at the country level. A username and a password are provided by WHO to each designated national rabies focal contact. Once validated by the WHO, data are transferred into Rabnet version 2. Username and password are not required to access or consult Rabnet data on human and animal rabies (WHO, 2008b). Rabnet keeps the same basic information resources containing ready-made maps, rabies-related documents, and details of collaborating centers. These data can be linked to a broad range of country-specific indicators (population, education, and health services) to provide a more comprehensive picture of the situation at different levels. This will help in understanding the disease prevalence and to formulate effective strategies for preventing the spread and occurrence of disease in various parts of the world.

WORLD RABIES DAY: "WORKING TOGETHER TO MAKE RABIES HISTORY!"

World Rabies Day (www.worldrabiesday.org) is an initiative of the Alliance for Rabies Control (ARC), co-founded by the CDC in Atlanta, Georgia, and supported by partners around the world, that is committed to its objective of raising global awareness and resources to enhance the prevention and control of rabies (World Rabies Day, 2008). The overall vision is successful human rabies prevention and

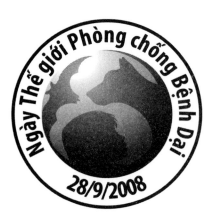

The logo of *World Rabies Day 2008* in Vietnamese.

elimination of dog-to-dog transmission of rabies. WHO and the Pan American Health Organization also supported this initiative. The inaugural World Rabies Day was organized on September 8, 2007, with the goal of building the political will necessary to end rabies. The ARC, CDC, World Organization for Animal Health, World Veterinary Association, World Society for the Protection of Animals, Pasteur Institute, Canadian Food Inspection Agency, Kansas State University, Association for the Control of Rabies in India, American Veterinary Medical Association, American Association of Animal Hospitals, British Veterinary Association, Commonwealth Veterinary Association, Student American Veterinary Association, National Association of State Public Health Veterinarians (U.S.), and Rabies in Asia Conference Foundation joined together in organizing the event. The initial goal was to mobilize 55,000 people, one for each person who dies from rabies each year worldwide. The inaugural campaign was a great success, engaging more than 393,000 people worldwide. Events were held in 74 countries. The mission statement was "Working Together to Make Rabies History!"

Several activities were planned to raise awareness of rabies in the campaign. School children in Thailand brought dogs to veterinary clinics for vaccination. Symposiums were held. Political leaders were contacted to raise the awareness and obtain funding for rabies-control measures. Several collaborators have joined to make the program a success. The CDC has organized communications and invitations to promote World Rabies Day. The U.S. Student American Veterinary Medical Association issued a challenge to chapters at colleges to plan World Rabies Day events. The Kansas State College of Veterinary Medicine prepared its first annual "Run 4 Rabies" in conjunction with World Rabies Day on September 8, 2007. The Pasteur Institute introduced the initiative to their international network of institutions. The Commonwealth Veterinary Association encouraged events at colleges of veterinary medicine throughout Asia. The Pan American Health Organization introduced the initiative to their member countries. Because of the success of the first World Rabies Day, a second world rabies day is planned for September 8, 2008. Although the major impact of rabies occurs in regions of the world where many other needs are present, rabies should no longer be neglected. The tools and technology for human rabies prevention and dog rabies elimination are available. Awareness of the problem and the political will of the participants are the typical limiting factors to achieve this goal.

ARC

Rabies is a neglected disease in vast parts of Asia and Africa. Children are particularly vulnerable to rabies: An estimated 100 youngsters below the age of 15 are dying around the globe every day because of rabies. It is well known that mass vaccination of stray dogs combined with an efficient postexposure treatment program is the most cost-effective way to control rabies. The developing world lacks the delivery systems, public education campaigns, and resources to apply these technologies. A team of international rabies experts met to consider the scale of the global rabies problem between 2003 and 2005. They recognized the need for a multidisciplinary group to focus efforts on combating this terrible disease. The ARC is the culmination of such efforts. ARC became a registered charity in the UK in January 2006. The ARC brings a new perspective to rabies control because it is not confined to the constraints of operating within governmental policies and procedures. ARC is an independent, nonprofit organization, bringing together public and private expertise in the field of rabies. ARC aims to involve medical, veterinary, wildlife, and animal welfare agencies to coordinate their rabies prevention efforts worldwide.

ARC successfully organized the first World Rabies Day. The ARC has identified Africa and Asia as priority areas because countries in these regions suffer the highest proportion of the world's human rabies burden and have the least capacity to combat this burden. They have created two advisory groups, one to provide advice on rabies programs and the other to provide advice on associated animal welfare and conservation issues. They have also instituted grant programs to encourage novel rabies control programs in the community in the developing world. ARC also provides opportunities for volunteers.

VETS BEYOND BORDERS

Vets Beyond Borders (VBB, previously known as Vetcharity) is an Australian-based, not-for-profit, incorporated organization established by veterinary volunteers in 2003. VBB is actively involved in the rabies control programs in Asia. VBB coordinates and runs veterinary-based animal welfare and public health programs in developing countries of Asia and the Pacific region (http://www.vetsbeyondborders.org). Emphasis is given to the training of local veterinary and paraveterinary staff to ensure that the work will continue. VBB relies on volunteers and promotes volunteer work amongst the veterinary community.

The overpopulation of street dogs is being addressed by VBB. WHO estimates there are more than 400 million stray dogs in the world today. They work with local governments to neuter street dogs and vaccinate them. This will result in the formation of a smaller, stable rabies-immune dog population. VBB is running two projects in India—The Sikkim Anti-Rabies and Animal Health (SARAH) program in partnership with the Government of Sikkim, and the Ladakh street dog project in partnership with the Ladakh Animal Care Society. Other voluntary organizations are also active in this area, especially in the developing world.

COSTS OF RABIES PREVENTION EFFORTS

It is very difficult to arrive at an accurate estimate of the total global costs to control and treat rabies. Although rabies has a low incidence in the developed world, the cost of rabies control can be enormous. Periodic vaccination of domestic animals and rabies-control strategies in the wild, including oral vaccines, are effective, but they are also costly. Postexposure prophylaxis can also become costly if several hundred people have been exposed. Such campaigns could easily add up to a million dollars in costs for each single episode. Although human rabies deaths are rare, the estimated public health costs associated with disease detection, prevention, and control have risen. The estimated cost of prevention of rabies is $230 million to $1 billion per year in the United States alone. These costs include the vaccination of companion animals, animal control programs, maintenance of rabies laboratories, and medical costs such as those incurred for rabies postexposure prophylaxis. This cost is shared by the private sector (primarily the vaccination of companion animals) and by the public (through animal control programs, maintenance of rabies laboratories, and subsidizing of rabies postexposure prophylaxis).

Accurate estimates of these expenditures are not available. Even in the richest countries, the cost of an effective dog rabies-control program is a drain on public health resources. An annual turnover of approximately 25 percent in the dog population necessitates revaccination of millions of animals each year.

The reintroduction of rabies through transport of infected animals from outside a controlled area is always a possibility should control programs lapse. Reservoirs of wildlife rabies are also potential sources of rabies infection for dogs in Europe and North America. Although the number of postexposure prophylaxes given in the United States each year is unknown, it is estimated to be around 40,000. When rabies becomes epizootic or enzootic in a region, the number of postexposure prophylaxes in that area increases. A course of rabies immune globulin and five doses of rabies vaccine given over a 4-week period typically exceeds $1,000. The cost per human life saved from rabies ranges from approximately $10,000 to $100 million, depending on the nature of the exposure and the probability of rabies in a region (CDC, 2008b).

Surveillance-related costs also rise as rabies becomes entrenched in wildlife. During 1993, the New York State Rabies Diagnostic Laboratory received approximately 12,000 suspected animal submissions. This compares with approximately 3,000 submissions in 1989, before raccoon rabies became epizootic. In New Jersey, rabies prevention expenditures in two counties increased from $768,488 in 1988, before the raccoon epizootic, to $1,952,014 in 1990, the first full year of the epizootic; vaccination of pet animals accounted for 82 percent of this total. Vaccinated domestic animals are normally administered a booster vaccine dose after a known or suspected rabid animal exposure. This increases costs further as wildlife rabies epizootics escalate.

$1.5 Million for Exposure to a Kitten

A case of rabies that occurred in New Hampshire attests to the potential high costs of rabies prevention. On October 24, 1994, the laboratory of the New Hampshire Division of Public Health Services (NHDPHS) diagnosed rabies in a kitten (CDC, 1995). This kitten was purchased from a pet store in Concord, New Hampshire. The animal developed seizures and died. Genetic typing of the rabies virus isolated from the kitten revealed close similarity with the raccoon variety of the virus. On October 12, a raccoon was captured from the suburbs of Concord where the kitten was suspected to have originated. This raccoon tested positive for rabies. Three other feral kittens acquired by the pet store were also thought to have contact with this raccoon. All three feral kittens developed signs of respiratory illness and died during approximately October 4–6. This was the time the original rabid kitten was in the store. The kittens were allowed to roam freely throughout the store, which was frequented by children from child-care centers and a nearby school. Local news media assisted in alerting the community residents about the potential exposures to rabies at the store. The health department screened approximately 1,000 persons who responded to media alerts and referred them to their medical providers. The medical providers were given guidelines to determine the eligibility of rabies postexposure prophylaxis. Rabies postexposure treatment consisted of one dose of rabies immune globulin and five doses of rabies vaccine. Approximately 665 persons received rabies postexposure prophylaxis because of exposure to this kitten and other cats from the same pet store. The overall estimated cost was $1.5 million, including expenditures for rabies immune globulin and vaccine ($1.1 million), laboratory testing of animals ($4,200), and investigation by NHDPHS and CDC personnel ($15,000).

Cost of Rabies in Developing Countries

Estimating the true costs of rabies in the developing world is complex. Despite evidence that the control of dog rabies through programs of animal vaccination and elimination of stray dogs can reduce the incidence of human rabies, exposure to rabid dogs is still the cause of more than 90 percent of human exposures to rabies and of more than 99 percent of human deaths from rabies worldwide. The cost of these programs prohibits their full implementation in much of the developing world. Worldwide, more than 7 million people receive postexposure prophylaxis yearly after being bitten by a rabid animal. In developing countries, treatment is not just expensive, but time consuming as well. A full course of vaccination requires five visits to a hospital or health clinic during one month. In rural Africa, this may need many hours of travel, time spent not working (Judson, 2008). Underreporting is a characteristic of almost every infectious disease in developing countries, so an accurate estimate of the costs may be impossible. Rabies is primarily not a human disease. It is primarily an animal disease and humans are the incidental victims. A more realistic estimate of the global burden of rabies should also take into account the impact on public health and the expense involved in preventing transmission of rabies from animals to humans.

Most economic analyses do not consider the human costs of the disease. These include the psychological trauma caused by human exposure to rabies, the subsequent euthanasia of pets, or the loss of wildlife resources during rabies outbreaks. Rabies incidence in wildlife is at an all-time high, and the cost of preventing this disease is steadily climbing (Rupprecht et al., 1995).

ROLE OF THE WHO IN RABIES PREVENTION EFFORTS

The WHO plays an important role in the worldwide control of rabies (WHO, 2008a). WHO actively supports several programs described earlier.

Customarily, the level of international resources committed to the control of an infectious disease is a response to the associated human morbidity and mortality. For most infectious diseases, these data adequately reflect the deserved public health attention. However, it is difficult to estimate the global impact of rabies by using only human mortality data. Most deaths from rabies occur in countries with inadequate public health resources and limited access to preventive treatment because effective vaccines to prevent human rabies have been available for more than 100 years. These countries also have few diagnostic facilities and almost no rabies surveillance. The total cost of rabies also includes control and vaccination efforts as well. WHO closely works with national health departments to coordinate effective rabies control programs, irrespective of the news value of the disease. It has produced several manuals on rabies control and set the standards worldwide. WHO has provided important insight into the control of stray dogs and rabies. Indiscriminate culling of stray dogs is not the best approach to controlling their population. ABC (Animal Birth Control) is the favored program for stray dog control. Several WHO documents provide guidelines for the national agencies to follow. WHO and WHO-collaborating centers and affiliated institutions cooperate with governments and national institutions to achieve these goals.

For rabies to be controlled, a sustained push is necessary. Improvement of the sociopolitical environment is also necessary for an effective rabies control program. The pervasiveness of rabies may be closely linked to other factors such as an unstable political system, level of education, national debts, and cultural beliefs in the developing nations. Rabies will probably never be eradicated totally from this world because of its widespread prevalence in wild animals and different terrestrial animals, including bats. A more realistic approach is to keep the rabies infections at an absolute minimum among domestic animals and humans. Any vaccination programs directed at animals should be perpetual; otherwise the offspring of those animals that are nonimmune can act as the new carriers of the disease.

7

The Current and Future Trends in Rabies

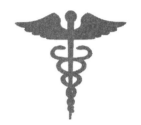

IS RABIES AN EMERGING DISEASE?

Rabies remains a major health problem because of its global distribution, and wide host range, including all mammals. The virus is maintained in nature by the sylvatic and urban cycles affecting different species. Once rabies is established in a particular species, disease transmission can persist for decades. This dynamic is obvious in the different epizootics of rabies in the United States. The spread of raccoon rabies along the East Coast from Florida to the northeast is an excellent example. Rabies is an emerging disease in this sense. *Emerging Infectious Diseases* is a scholarly journal addressing the advent of new diseases worldwide that also publishes research papers on rabies. This journal is published by the Centers for Disease Control and Prevention (CDC) in Atlanta, Georgia.

Rabies virus is the most important species of the genus *Lyssavirus*. Unlike rabies, distribution of the six other lyssaviruses is much more limited, and little is known about their host range. Only select hosts can carry each of these genotypes. They also seem to cause only endemic levels of transmission. Only six deaths have been reported so far in association with the six *Lyssavirus* genotypes. However, it is likely that several infections caused by these viruses may go undiagnosed because of low awareness. The exact health implications of the lyssaviruses are unknown. It is possible that newly found viruses may be added to this group in the future. The seventh serotype of *Lyssavirus* was most recently detected in Australia. Australia used to be a rabies- (and *Lyssavirus-*) free continent. *Lyssavirus* is a re-emerging threat to animal and human health all over the world. An increase of rabies in wildlife has led to the development of vaccines for oral administration. Safe human rabies vaccines are highly expensive. Vaccines of high immunogenicity that are safe, easily produced, and have an extended protection period are needed worldwide. For these reasons, constant research is being done to improve understanding of the disease and help find new methods of prevention and immunization.

Bat Rabies as an Emerging Zoonosis

Bat variants of the rabies virus are of increasing public health importance worldwide. Bat-associated rabies has become the predominant form of rabies seen in the United States. Bats are the reservoir and vector for six out of the seven genotypes of the lyssaviruses characterized so far. Four recent isolates of Asian bat lyssaviruses are proposed as new genotypes, and new isolates from bats are expected. The World Health Organization (WHO) recommends future research on the different lyssaviruses in bats, and the risk to humans. Existing bat rabies data need to be updated periodically. Areas of future research in this field include (1) active and passive surveillance of bat rabies, (2) molecular epidemiology and antigenic profile of bat *Lyssavirus* isolates throughout Eurasia, (3) identification of spillover infections, and (4) studies on the pathogenicity of those viruses on bats and other terrestrial animals. Spillover infection into terrestrial animals from bats is a possibility, although not reported so far.

In this evolving scenario, public awareness needs to be increased about the new dangers lurking around one's own home. This has to be done without invoking paranoia and panic. The presence of an effective vaccine in the case of rabies might instill confidence in the general public unlike other devastating viral infections, such as Ebola, that have no vaccine. However, the history of rabies lives with us. The frightening picture of madness and a painful death is associated with each case report of rabies. Still, rabies is very uncommon in most parts of the world. On an average, two or three people die every year in the United States because of rabies. This pales in comparison to thousands dying each year of heart disease and cancers. Increased awareness among the public is needed to stop the emergence and spread of unusual infections such as rabies in the developed world. The Massachusetts Department of Health in the United States has chronicled a cornucopia of stories to illustrate the challenges posed by the spread of rabies in terrestrial animals of the eastern United States and how a casual approach can worsen the situation.

LIVING WITH RABIES IN YOUR COMMUNITY: MASSACHUSETTS DEPARTMENT OF PUBLIC HEALTH, 2002–2004

Raccoon rabies spread from the southeastern United States and along the eastern Atlantic coast, reaching Massachusetts in 1992. The Massachusetts Department of Public Health has published interesting episodes in which people have unknowingly come into contact with rabies. These vignettes are aimed to raise the awareness of rabies among the public. They also illustrate the efforts by the department to control and contain the rabies cases. These cases are based on reports to the department between 2002 and 2004. The state coordinated the efforts, but the exposed individual and his/her primary care physician decided about rabies postexposure prophylaxis (Massachusetts Department of Public Health, 2004).

Road Kill in a School Refrigerator

Norfolk County, Raccoon

One of the teachers at the local school found a dead raccoon on the side of the road and placed it in the school refrigerator for future dissection in a biology class. A custodian spotted the dead animal in the refrigerator and the health department was alerted. Fortunately, there was no exposure to the raccoon and no one needed any prophylaxis. Subsequently, the school developed policies regarding appropriate subjects for biology class demonstrations. It was not known whether the raccoon was rabid.

Cows Are at Risk of Rabies

Plymouth County, Cow

A farmer in Plymouth County noticed two calves having weakness, buckling, and shaking of the hind legs. Shortly after, they were unable to stand, although they continued to eat and remained alert. The calves died 7 days after the onset of the illness. They later tested positive for rabies. The calves were unvaccinated against rabies. Several feral cats and one skunk had been spotted around the barn. Another calf that was with the two calves was quarantined for 6 months and then found to be healthy. There were 130 adult cows in the herd but none were vaccinated against rabies. They were recommended rabies vaccinations. The farm owner, his wife, the veterinarian, three workers on the farm, and a family friend and her two children received postexposure prophylaxis.

Danger of House Animals Outdoors Before They Can Be Vaccinated

Norfolk County, Dog

A 14-week-old female boxer puppy developed progressive neurological symptoms. The animal's condition worsened over the next few days and it had to be put to sleep. The puppy tested positive for rabies. Further investigations revealed that the puppy was purchased from a private home. The mother had seven puppies and was caged outdoors. A skunk was spotted with the mother and the puppies in the cage one day. The department advised strict 6 months of confinement for the rest of the puppies in the litter. Staff of the three animal hospitals where the puppy was treated received postexposure rabies prophylaxis. It was also discovered that a few days before the puppy was ill it had been transported in a ferry. The health department contacted each passenger on the list provided by the ferry company and they were contacted by the health department for any potential exposure to the puppy. About 22 individuals received postexposure prophylaxis.

No Live Demonstrations with Dead Animals!

Essex County, Coyote

A carpentry teacher saw a dead coyote on the side of the road and gave a skinning demonstration to a group of 13 students at a local high school. None of them wore gloves. It was thought that the students might have had contacts with the saliva of the dead animal. Rabies testing could not be done because of the condition of the specimen. At the school, rumors were circulating about what was done to the coyote and where the animal had been in the school. This made it difficult to determine who had been exposed. A letter was sent to 420 parents and staff to notify them of the incident and to find the people who had been exposed. The authorities did not take any chances and two students received postexposure prophylaxis. The teacher was suspended by the school administration following the incident.

Rabid Raccoon Entering a House through a "Doggy Door"

Middlesex County, Raccoon

A raccoon came inside a house through a doggy door while the homeowners were away. A pet sitter arrived at the house later to take care of the two pet dogs but found blood all over the house. The smaller dog had been mauled to death in the bedroom. The raccoon was still in the room, so the animal control officer was called. The officer killed the raccoon and the specimen was submitted for rabies testing. The second dog survived, but was bitten by the raccoon. This dog was up to date with rabies vaccines and was given a booster dose, and the pet sitter started postexposure prophylaxis for indirect exposure. The rabies tests were positive in the raccoon.

Skunks Attack Puppy in the Back Yard

Plymouth County, Dog

A skunk attacked a 10-week-old puppy in the owner's yard a few feet from their door. The puppy did not have any visible wounds. The family members comforted the puppy by holding and petting it. The skunk could not be located for testing. Five family members were given rabies postexposure prophylaxis because they may have had indirect exposure to the skunk through contact with its saliva on the puppy. The puppy had not been vaccinated against rabies because of his young age. The family was given the option of either putting the puppy to sleep or to quarantine him for 6 months. The family decided to quarantine the puppy. The puppy was only allowed to have limited contact with adult family members and could only go outside to go to the bathroom. Unfortunately, 6 weeks later the puppy developed neurological signs suggestive of rabies. He was brought to a veterinarian who put him to sleep and submitted his head for rabies testing. The puppy tested positive for rabies.

Wild Fox under the Porch

Middlesex County, Fox

A fox and her litter of puppies were living underneath the porch of a resident. A neighbor saw this and tried to take a picture. The mother fox bit the neighbor. The fox was submitted for rabies testing and tested positive. The neighbor was given rabies postexposure prophylaxis. A pet cat exposed to the fox was up to date with rabies vaccinations. A booster dose was given to the cat. The cat was quarantined for 45 days. The animal control officer was notified about the positive rabies test in the fox, and the fox puppies living underneath the porch were put to sleep.

Rabies Danger of Feral Cats

Essex County, Massachusetts, Cat

A kitten was living with about 15 feral cats (unowned stray cats) in a barn. The owner of the barn wanted to evacuate these animals. Foster families took most of the cats before permanent homes were found for them. A foster family cared for the kitten for 2 months. A second family adopted the kitten but the kitten was injured from a fall from a window. A veterinarian recommended that the kitten be put to sleep because of the severe injuries it sustained. The kitten had recently bitten its owner, hence it was submitted for rabies testing. The kitten tested positive for rabies. Both families received postexposure rabies prophylaxis. The second family also had two other cats obtained from the same barn. These cats had been in close contact with the rabid kitten. The family was encouraged either to have these two cats put to sleep and submitted for testing or to quarantine them for 6 months.

SCIENTIFIC RESEARCH IN RABIES AND THE FUTURE

Research in rabies has mainly focused upon developing better vaccines and increasing the efficacy of the available vaccines. The initial vaccines discovered by Pasteur were based on animal neural tissue and carried a high incidence of complications. These neural vaccines are being phased out all over the world with the advent of the human diploid cell strain vaccine that carries far fewer complications. Newer technologies are being derived to increase the efficacy of the vaccines.

The essential goal for rabies vaccine development is the invention of safe, portable, and inexpensive vaccines. Although vaccine strategies have greatly reduced the disease burden in developed countries, programs to vaccinate wild and domestic animals are the key to continuing these trends. Possible candidates for a future vaccine include an avirulent escape mutant SAG-2 that may be used for animal vaccination. This mutant virus is avirulent (nonvirulent) in rodents, cats, dogs, and foxes, yet gives immunological protection from virulent strains. Other possibilities for new vaccines include edible plant vaccines expressing rabies antigens. Recombinant plant viruses such as tobacco mosaic virus could also be modified to deliver important epitopes encoding genes to elicit a protective immune response. An epitope is a small portion of a larger protein or organism recognized by the body's immune system. Such epitopes can be introduced into a virus such as tobacco mosaic virus through recombination.

Safety Precautions in Research

As we make more progress towards controlling rabies worldwide, it is very important to focus on the safety of rabies virus research. All persons involved in rabies testing should receive pre-exposure immunization with regular serologic tests and booster immunizations as necessary. Unimmunized individuals should not enter laboratories where rabies work is conducted. All tissues processed in an infectious disease laboratory must be disposed of as medical waste. All activities related to the handling of animals and samples for rabies diagnosis should be performed using appropriate biosafety practices to avoid direct contact with potentially infected tissues. The CDC has designated four levels of safety, or biosafety levels (BSLs). Different diseases require work at different levels of safety (CDC, 2000). BSL 1 is suitable for work involving well-characterized organisms that are not known to cause disease in normal healthy individuals. BSL 2 involves organisms with slightly more risk. The personnel are better trained and special precautions are taken to avoid contamination with sharp objects or aerosols. The next level, BSL 3, is used when research is done on indigenous or exotic agents that may cause serious or potentially lethal disease if exposed through the inhalation route. Examples include anthrax, West Nile virus, Venezuelan equine encephalitis, eastern equine encephalitis, SARS (severe acute respiratory syndrome), tuberculosis, typhus, Rift Valley fever, Rocky Mountain spotted fever, and yellow fever. Although these diseases could be fatal if contracted by a worker, vaccines and other types of treatment might exist for them. The exhaust from the laboratory is discarded outside so that any aerosols are eliminated from the environment around the researchers. BSL 4 is required for work with the most dangerous and exotic infective agents. The examples include Bolivian and Argentine hemorrhagic fevers, smallpox, Marburg virus, Ebola virus, Hanta virus, Lassa fever, and Crimean-Congo hemorrhagic fever. These infective agents pose the highest level of danger and risk of transmission by aerosols. A hazmat suit and a self-contained oxygen supply are mandatory for BSL 4 workers. The entrance and exits should contain multiple showers, a vacuum room, an ultraviolet light room, and other safety precautions for decontamination. A rabies laboratory is generally BSL 2. Some rabies research is done at BSL 3.

Personnel working in rabies laboratories are at risk of rabies infection through accidental injection or contamination of mucous membranes with rabies virus-contaminated material and also by exposure to aerosols of rabies-infected material. All manipulations of tissues and slides should be conducted in a manner that does not aerosolize liquids or produce airborne particles. Barrier protection is required for safe removal of brain tissue from animals submitted for rabies testing. At a minimum, barrier protection during necropsy should include the following as personal protective equipment (PPE): heavy rubber gloves, laboratory gown and waterproof apron, boots, surgical masks, protective sleeves, and a face shield. Fume hoods or biosafety hoods are not required, but they provide additional protection from odor, ectoparasites, and bone fragments. Glass chips and shards from slide manipulations are also potential sources of exposure to rabies. Care should be taken to protect eyes and hands during the manipulation and staining of slides and during cleanup of the microscope and surrounding area. A special microscope adaptor is available to provide eye protection from any glass splinters produced when slides are moved across the microscope stage. Ergonomic equipment (fatigue mat, microscope controls) should be used to prevent fatigue-related injuries to employees during lengthy necropsy and slide-reading procedures (CDC, 2008c).

Genetic Vaccine for Rabies

This is a novel idea to use only part of the genome for designing a vaccine against an infective agent. Adenovirus is ubiquitous and adenoviral infections in humans are common. Respiratory tract diseases such as the common cold, pneumonia, and bronchitis; disease of the intestines such as diarrhea; and conjunctivitis of eyes are commonly caused by adenovirus. Because of its high infectivity, researchers have used adenovirus as vectors (carriers) of different genes in gene therapy studies or vaccine trials. One strategy is to piggyback the rabies virus genetic code into a defective adenovirus. The idea here is twofold. By using only the genetic code of the rabies that codes for the rabies antigen, the researchers aimed to bombard the healthy person with an antigen that will evoke maximum immune response. Because this is not the whole rabies virus, complications are less.

The adenovirus is made defective by deliberately deleting some of its genes so that these viruses cannot replicate independently in human beings. Researchers thought that using a chimpanzee strain of the adenovirus as the vector would be more successful because most people are infected by adenovirus during childhood and carry significant antibody titers. These persons may be immune to the adenovirus and subsequently may not become infected with the vaccine. Hence, the researchers used a simian adenoviral vector derived from a chimpanzee isolate. These viruses do not circulate in the human population and do not cross-react with the common human adenoviruses. Manufacturing such a vaccine is a delicate process. The simian adenoviral vector termed adenovirus C68 (AdC68) was produced initially. The full-length coding sequence for the glycoprotein of rabies virus was isolated and fixed to this adenoviral vector in a particular spot. This molecular engineering technique is known as recombination. Once this recombinant vaccine gets into the recipient's body, the genes coding for the glycoprotein part of the rabies virus will stimulate the production of specific antibodies that will protect the human beings from rabies. Several researchers have performed successful animal experiments on this topic. For example, Dr. Xiang and colleagues proved that such a vaccine injected into mice made them immune to rabies. They were not sickened by fatal doses of rabies virus. (Xiang, et al., 2002). In mice, this vaccine induced complete protection from rabies after a single injection.

Adenovirus-based vaccines are not ready for primetime yet. Scientists are still working on the technical details. Several tragedies such as deaths of volunteers that happened during various gene therapy trials using these vectors prompted tighter scrutiny. Oral and mucosal delivery forms are also being tested in animals. These routes offer significant promise in the rabies-control field because this type of vaccine may be easier for developing countries to obtain. Vector-associated vaccines can impart complete protection from rabies virus after a single dose.

New Technology for Oral Rabies Vaccine

Oral rabies vaccines are currently used to immunize wild animals against rabies. They are dispersed with baits either terrestrially or aerially from an aircraft or helicopter. Researchers from Thomas Jefferson University are working on another way to produce oral vaccines for wild animals. They manipulated the rabies virus itself, making it much weaker. This vaccine is much more immunogenic because it has the live virus incorporated. Live vaccines always have the potential to transmit the disease they are intended to prevent. This danger was minimized in the vaccine and the lack of pathogenicity was proven in several mice experiments. Using "bioreactor technology" in a sophisticated cell culture system, scientists are able to produce large quantities of the vaccine relatively fast and inexpensively, which is an added benefit of this new type of oral vaccine. Again, no human oral vaccines are available now.

Tobacco Plant as a Vaccine Factory

The idea of using the tobacco plant to produce massive quantities of oral anti-rabies vaccine is an exciting new development in vaccine research. The idea is to use the plants as vaccine factories. Plant viruses such as tobacco mosaic virus (TMV) and tomato bushy virus can be used as vectors. The rabies genes that codes for the different proteins of the virus are inserted into the proper areas of the vector virus (Jackson and Wunner, 2002, 389). The tobacco plant is still being investigated as a suitable plant factory for this purpose. The recombinant plant viruses infect and multiply in the plants, and large amounts of oral vaccines could be produced by these multiplying viruses. This method is still in the experimental stage, but holds significant promises in vaccine production.

Monoclonal Antibodies

Monoclonal antibodies are one of the latest advances in rabies. They are meant to replace the rabies immune globulin (RIG) of human or equine origin. Both products have risks of infection or allergies. Any antigens, which include viruses, stimulate the production of antibodies in the body. Monoclonal antibodies are very specific "magic bullets" directed against only one type of antigen. Monoclonal antibodies are used to treat various ailments such as cancer, cardiovascular disease, inflammatory diseases, macular degeneration, transplant rejection, and multiple sclerosis. With rabies, this method is still in the experimental stages. Usually monoclonal antibodies are produced with the help of mouse cells. Being foreign cells, a mouse-cell-derived monoclonal antibody can produce reactions in humans. To circumvent this, a method called humanization of the monoclonal antibody is adopted. In one approach, DNA coding for a protein from mice is fused with human DNA in the laboratory, and this combined DNA is injected into mammalian cell cultures to produce the antibodies. These "humanized" antibodies are better tolerated with fewer complications.

Several researchers and manufacturers are going through different trials of rabies monoclonal antibody that is humanized. Molecular Targeting Technologies, Inc., is a privately held biotechnology company located in West Chester, Pennsylvania. The company is working with the North China Pharmaceutical Group Corporation (NCPC), with headquarters in Shijiazhuang, to develop a human antirabies monoclonal antibody (Mab) product in China for postexposure treatment of rabies (Molecular Targeting Technologies, 2008). Another Mab initially developed at the Thomas Jefferson University (TJU) in Philadelphia was shown to neutralize a wide variety of strains of rabies. This will help in the usage of this antibody in different parts of the world, and in rabies found in several wild animals. These antibodies are produced through cell culture technologies and are a serum-free rabies Mab product that is free from potential contamination with human pathogens.

Another manufacturer, Crucell, also has developed a human Mab cocktail in collaboration with TJU in Philadelphia and the CDC in Atlanta (Crucell, 2006). Multiple phase 1 studies were carried out in the United States in 2006 and in Asia during 2007. Crucell and Sanofi Pasteur signed an exclusive collaboration and commercialization agreement for the development of a rabies Mab cocktail, using Crucell's manufacturing technology. This antibody cocktail is to be used with the rabies vaccine for postexposure prophylaxis against this fatal disease.

After the encouraging U.S. phase 1 study, Crucell conducted a phase 1b study in India with the antibody cocktail. They found that that the cocktail is well tolerated, provides the expected neutralizing activity, and can be safely administered in combination with a rabies vaccine. Because of these studies, the Food and Drug Administration (FDA) has given a fast-track designation for this Mab. Under the terms of the agreement, Crucell will continue to perform the development activities. Crucell will be responsible for the manufacturing of the final product and will retain exclusive distribution rights in Europe, co-exclusive distribution rights in China, and the rights to sell to supranational organizations such as UNICEF. In the open part of the phase 1b trial, rabies Mab cocktail was administered in combination with a rabies vaccine; all volunteers seroconverted within 14 days upon initiation of treatment. A level of rabies virus neutralizing activity (>0.5 IU/mL) was achieved in all cases. This level is considered to give protection against rabies. It was also proven that the antibody cocktail can be safely administered along with the standard treatment with vaccines.

Virus Identification Using Mabs

Mabs are also being investigated as a diagnostic tool in rabies. Mabs for rabies diagnostic purposes are produced by a mouse-myeloma cell combination known as hybridoma. These hybridoma cells are injected with either rabies or rabies-related viruses. These hybridomas then secrete Mabs directed against the glycoprotein (G protein) that is a part of the covering of the rabies virus.

Specific antibodies can be produced in this manner, targeting a special variant of the virus. This will also help in characterizing the type of the virus isolated. Different panels of Mabs can be used to differentiate the rabies virus isolates from terrestrial and bat host species in the United States, western Europe, and, to a lesser extent in Africa, Asia, eastern Europe, and Latin America. WHO coordinated these efforts between 1982 and 1990 and two panels of Mabs have been established to identify various *Lyssavirus* serotypes (WHO, 2008c). This panel is also used in the differentiation of major virus strains used for vaccine production from field virus isolates. Currently, Mabs are used mainly for epidemiological and research purposes. They do not have a significant role in the routine diagnosis of rabies yet, despite their early promise.

Tobacco Plant to Produce Antibodies against Rabies

Recent advances in molecular biology and plant biotechnology have raised the potential for using plants as factories for the production of therapeutic recombinant proteins. This is beyond the traditional plant cultivation aimed at producing food crops. Plants could be versatile "biopharming factories" because they are capable of producing large amounts of recombinant proteins safely and inexpensively. An effective plant production system for recombinant biologicals will have multiple components. These include an appropriate plant expression system, optimal combination of gene expression and regulatory elements, control of the processing of the product by the plant, and efficient purification methods for product recovery. Scientists at TJU Medical College in Philadelphia have manipulated tobacco plants to produce rabies Mabs as well (Science Daily, 2003). This is a remarkable feat. A team of scientists led by Dr. Hilary Koprowski, a professor of microbiology and immunology, has succeeded in inserting DNA codes into tobacco plants. The genes they selected code for an antibody against the rabies virus. The plants in turn become plant factories churning out the antibodies. The worldwide shortage of antirabies biologicals can be abated by such a technology because transgenic plants have proven to be an efficient production system for the expression of functional therapeutic proteins when compared with conventional methods. Plant-derived Mabs have many advantages, such as the lack of animal pathogenic contaminants, a low cost of production, and ease of massive scale of production. Researchers have also shown that plant-derived antibody can neutralize rabies virus and prevent infection in mice. Using plant-derived antibody, researchers have also prevented rabies in hamsters inoculated with a lethal dose of rabies virus.

DNA Vaccines

DNA vaccines are the latest strategy for a new rabies vaccine. These vaccines, once developed, should offer immunizations that are both safer and cheaper than conventional vaccines. DNA vaccination differs from traditional vaccines in that only the DNA coding for a specific component of a disease-causing organism is injected into the body (Henahan, 1997). DNA vaccines use the smallest amount of genetic material from the virus to activate the immune system.

Vaccine Design

Researchers use plasmids for the construction of DNA vaccines. Plasmids are small circular DNAs that can replicate in bacteria. A suitable plasmid is selected first. DNA vaccines utilize naked DNA strands alone for immunization, without traditional proteins or carrier viruses. The genes encoding specific immunogenic proteins are inserted into a plasmid. This is accomplished using recombinant DNA technology. These vaccines elicit the best immunological response when they have a certain structure. Plasmids that have a string promoter gene will make the antibody production stronger. A region called intron A is also included in the plasmid vaccines. Once such a recombinant plasmid is constructed, it can be inserted into a bacterium. The growth and multiplication of the bacteria produces several copies of the plasmid DNA. This small circular plasmid DNA is purified from the larger bacterial cell DNA. The purified product is the DNA vaccine. Other elements introduced into the vaccine include the promoter gene, enhancer sequences, synthetic introns, and adenovirus tripartite leader (TPL) sequences.

Vaccine Delivery

A DNA vaccine is delivered directly into the cell. The actual production of the immunizing protein takes place in the vaccinated host. This eliminates any risk of infection that is associated with some live and attenuated virus vaccines. If delivered to the target cells directly, DNA can induce the host cells to produce chemicals to fight off the infection. Unfortunately, the delivery of DNA to target cells is still inefficient and undergoing research at this time. Several nuances of the technique including the type and characteristics of the carrier molecules and the modifications to be made on their genetic makeup are under investigation. DNA-based vaccines could be versatile because they can theoretically induce immunity through a wide variety of pathways. Different modes of delivery are being investigated apart from the traditional intramuscular or intradermal delivery. A unique system being explored is using a "gene gun." Rapid delivery of the DNA vaccine directly into the cells is achieved by using gene guns. This method of direct intracellular epidermal delivery consists of propelling DNA-coated gold beads through the plasma membrane of the cells. The cells are transected by these DNA molecules without invoking a cellular mechanism to swallow them. A booster dose of this type of vaccine can give rise to a strong antibody response because the cells "remember" the previous DNA shot. The major problem with these vaccines is the delayed first response in mounting an antibody response. The DNA vaccine approach holds considerable promises in rabies research. DNA vaccines have the following advantages over a conventional vaccine (American Society of Microbiology, 1997).

1. They provide long-lasting immunity and a single inoculation can confer prolonged immunity.
2. They might be effective against multiple infections and can replace vaccines that are given over a lengthy period of time such as multiple childhood immunizations.
3. The production of the vaccine may be simpler and also more sophisticated.
4. They are much safer without any contamination of blood, blood products, or other antigens. The chance of an accidental infection occurring is almost zero because only part of the DNA is used for the vaccine production.
5. The immunity imparted to the individual can be very focused to a particular infection.

6. They can be produced by simple techniques in large amounts.
7. They are extremely stable. This is important in developing countries where the cold chain of vaccines may not maintained because of economic or power supply problems. Cold chain is the usage of a series of refrigerators to keep the vaccine cold and effective during its transportation from the point of manufacturing to the place of immunization. The lack of such a chain can dramatically reduce the efficacy of a vaccine.
8. Vaccines can be designed faster to counter newly evolving diseases. The DNA needed for developing the vaccine can be directly isolated from the infected animal or human being.
9. They are much more cost-effective than traditional vaccines. This increases their affordability in developing countries.

The disadvantages of the DNA vaccines are:

1. This method is limited to developing immune responses only against the protein components of pathogens.
2. The ideal vector for such a vaccine is still debated. Some of the viral vectors used in clinical studies have had untoward effects, such as adenoviral vectors used in the gene therapy trials.
3. The outer walls of some of the infecting organism are made up of polymerized sugars, known as polysaccharides. DNA vaccines cannot substitute for the more traditional polysaccharide-based vaccines. The pneumococcal vaccine used to prevent bacterial pneumonia is an example.
4. The delay in mounting an effective immunity can be lengthy.
5. Various safety issues are being raised about the DNA vaccines. The inserted genetic material of the DNA vaccine might integrate with the cellular DNA and provoke untoward effects such as cancer.
6. The development of autoimmunity (the body fighting against itself) is another early concern about DNA vaccines.
7. The plasmid vectors used in the formulation of vaccines are cultured in an antibiotic-resistant milieu. One of the early fears was that this might cause the spread of antibiotic resistance. This turned out to be not true, because the bacterial resistance is confined strictly to the bacterial cells and not the mammalian cells. The recipients of a DNA vaccine remain unaffected.

Apart from the buzz, there are only a few successful trials of the DNA vaccines so far. Rabies is not among them. A DNA vaccine for bird flu showed some promise in 2006. A veterinary DNA vaccine to protect horses from West Nile virus was also approved. Another preliminary study of a DNA vaccine in multiple sclerosis offered some promise. On the contrary, much-touted DNA vaccines for diseases seen worldwide such as AIDS and malaria have not been successful as of yet.

Rabies Virus for Vaccines against Other Viruses

An interesting spin-off of research with the rabies virus is its use in vaccines against other viral diseases. Rabies virus is being used to engineer a vaccine against simian immunodeficiency virus, a disease closely related to human AIDS. Researchers followed two steps in producing such a vaccine. First, they made the rabies virus incapable of multiplication by knocking out some of its genes essentially required for this purpose. Then they inserted parts of other viruses that can produce an antibody response in the body. More than 50 percent of a vector can be loaded with foreign antigens in this manner. Although this strategy was tested successfully in experimental animals, human experiments are yet to be conducted.

Rabies Receptors

Receptors are specialized molecules present on cell membranes. They are capable of binding to specific antigens or particles in a "lock-and-key" fashion. After attaching to the receptor, the receptor-antigen complex is formed and the cell internalizes the complex. The receptor usually empties the antigen or particle to the inside of the cells. This is an ingenious way of imbibing substances from the environment adopted by the cells. This activity can be seen in several single-cell organisms as well. After being introduced into the body by a biting animal, the free rabies virus seeks out the peripheral nerve endings. The rabies virus enters the peripheral nerves through receptors known as nicotinic acetylcholine receptors. Acetylcholine receptors are ion channels that span the neuronal membrane. They have three different portions—extracellular (outside the cell), intramembranous (inside the cell membrane), and cytoplasmic (inside the cell). They have five subunits arranged around a central ion channel. These receptors usually respond to the chemical substance secreted by some nerve endings known as acetylcholine. Acetylcholine is a chemical important in the communication between different nerve fibers in the body as well as muscle contractions. Once inside the nerve cells, the virus can slowly propagate through the nerve fibers until it reaches the brain. However, the rabies virus has the ability to infect several cell lines that do not express the acetylcholine receptor, suggesting that there are multiple receptors for the rabies virus.

The exact pathophysiology of rabies in the brain is unknown. Although rabies affects certain specific parts of the brain, often the clinical features are out of proportion to the damage visualized in the brain at autopsy. This prompted scientists to believe that the major pathological changes of rabies could be caused by the disturbance of neurotransmitters. Neurotransmitters are the chemicals important in the communication between the brain nerve cells. Rabies is also thought to bind with acetylcholine receptors in the brain. If this happens, it will block the normal actions of the acetylcholine because the rabies virus already occupies the receptor. This can lead to profound changes in brain function by disrupting the transmission of signals among brain cells (neurons).

The identification of specific rabies receptors will help in understanding the mechanism of infection in rabies. Rabies is known to infect neurons and lymphocytes. These cells have common surface molecules, specifically cytokine and chemokine receptors and adhesion molecules. Adhesion molecules have been reported to allow other viruses and parasites to infect these cells. The virus is also thought to use different receptors in the brain. Researchers examined the surface molecules of rabies-susceptible and nonsusceptible cell lines. Neural Cell Adhesion Molecule (NCAM) was found on the surface of all cell lines susceptible to rabies virus infection, but was not found on the surface of any resistant cell lines (Schweighardt and Atwood, 2001). NCAM is also called CD56. Experiments done in NCAM-deficient mice showed that the animals still died, despite the lack of NCAM. This means that the rabies virus in fact utilizes more than one receptor. Research provides strong evidence that NCAM plays a significant role as a receptor for rabies. A specific amino acid (333) in the G protein of rabies virus is also thought to play an important part in the binding of the virus to the NCAM receptor. When this amino acid is altered in the laboratory, the resulting virus is incapable of infecting other neurons. When this altered virus was inoculated into the nasal mucosa of experimental animals, only a few neurons were infected with the virus.

Another receptor implicated in the spread of infection by rabies virus is the low-affinity p75 neurotropic receptor. It is also called the nerve growth factor (NGF) receptor. Experiments with this receptor also demonstrated that this is not the only receptor used by rabies virus to gain entrance to the neural cells. Investigators were able to infect mice deficient in this receptor with rabies virus. These experiments suggest that rabies virus probably utilizes a wide array of receptors to gain access to the nervous system. Several companies and researchers are aiming to formulate a drug out of these receptors, but have not yet been successful because the detailed structure and characteristics of the receptors are unknown.

Neurotransmitters

Another hot field of research in rabies deals with the role of different chemicals in the brain. These chemicals are collectively known as neurotransmitters and act as the messengers for communication between various neuronal cells. Normal brain function and cognition is possible because of the actions of this intricate network. The full details of these systems are unknown at the present time although a large body of knowledge has been unraveled by years of research. Acetylcholine is thought to play an important role in the pathogenesis of rabies in the brain. Some of the research does cast doubt on this assertion, indicating that no single neurotransmitter may be at fault in rabies. Serotonin is another brain chemical thought to be important in the pathogenesis of rabies. Serotonin has important functions in the control of sleep and wakefulness, pain perception, memory, and a variety of behaviors. Some experiments in animals have suggested that rabies infection in the brain directly affects the receptors of serotonin. Some of these changes occur before the rabies virus enters the brain. Hence it is also possible that these changes could be due to an unknown mechanism triggered by the rabies virus infecting other parts of the body, before the virus reaches the brain. Gamma amino butyric acid (GABA) is another chemical suspected to be affected in rabies. Impairment in both the release and uptake of this chemical has been noted in the rat brain affected with rabies (Ladogana et al., 1994).

Ion Channels

Ion channels are present in every cell. They are small porous structures in the cell membrane directing the flow of ions into and out of the cell. They are voltage dependent and maintain a constant composition of different ions and chemicals inside the cell. Normal cellular function is tightly linked to a healthy ion channel system. Viral infections such as rabies could have profound effects on the ion channel. Some of the research does suggest a role for ion channel malfunction as the cause of the pathophysiological features of rabies. The hyperexcitability and aggressive behavior seen in rabies could be partially attributed to the malfunction of ion channels.

Apoptosis

Cells die physiologically in response to a variety of stimuli; this collective process is called apoptosis, or programmed cell death. This is a fascinating event occurring in any living organism in a coordinated fashion. Once the stimulus is triggered, a cell will deteriorate slowly. The cell membrane will lose its asymmetry and attachment. The cell shrinks and the nuclear material condenses. The nuclear material fragments, and these fragments are ingested by the phagocytes in the body. Apoptosis is characterized by the absence of an inflammatory reaction, unless there is necrosis of cells and tissue. Various stimuli can trigger apoptosis. The signals can either come from inside the cell or outside the cell. Apoptosis is likely to be an important role in several viral infections (Licata and Harty, 2003). Recent studies have demonstrated apoptosis of neurons in the rabies infected brain of mice in laboratory experiments. The presence of such neurons can be identified by special staining in the laboratory. However, not all infected cells show special staining suggestive of apoptosis. Apoptosis was more evident in the suckling mouse infected with rabies than in adult-infected mice. Apoptosis was reported in several experimental rabies infections in animals. Reports of apoptosis in naturally infected animals or humans are rare.

Nitric Oxide

Nitric oxide is another ubiquitous chemical important in several functions in different organs. Nitric oxide is a free radical and acts as the mediator of the phagocytic activity of the macrophages in mice. This helps in the fight with various bacterial, fungal, and viral pathogens. Nitric oxide has been shown to inhibit replication, helping in the clearance of certain viruses. Researchers have also postulated that nitric oxide might even be toxic to the brain cells. Some studies have proven that there are increasing quantities of nitrous oxide in experimental animals infected with rabies. The nitric oxide levels increased proportionately to the severity of symptoms. Nitric oxide formed by the macrophage may be toxic to the delicate neurons because nitric oxide can form harmful chemicals in combination with other substances present in the brain. The exact role of nitric oxide in rabies is unknown. It has both beneficial and deleterious effects. This topic deserves further study.

Antiviral Medications

Antiviral medications are different from antibiotics and other drugs effective against the usual bacterial infections such as pneumonia or skin infections. Antibiotics are not effective against viruses because viruses usually surreptitiously proliferate inside the cells. Antiviral drugs are far fewer in number than antibiotics. They target different stages of viral entry into the cell or enzymes involved in its multiplication to stop the viral multiplication. Viruses are smaller than bacteria and the exact mechanism by which the virus infects cells is unknown. Rabies researchers hope to design effective antiviral drugs once the exact mechanism by which rabies causes the pathological changes in the brain is known. Of the currently available drugs, ribavirin is believed to have some antiviral effects against rabies. Ribavirin is a broad spectrum antiviral drug and is effective against a wide variety of RNA viruses. It was used in the treatment of the Wisconsin teenager infected with rabies. However, several subsequent cases did not survive despite using this drug. It is doubtful that ribavirin is effective against rabies as a single agent. It might be useful as a part of a cocktail against rabies.

French researchers have reported the discovery of a new lyssavirus-based antiviral drug (Real et al., 2004). They identified phosphoprotein (P) as the prime target for inhibitors of viral replication. In this exhaustive method, two peptides were selected according to how they bind to the target protein, and the peptides were then tested for efficacy.

Another novel method proposed is known as biomimetic technology. NanoViricides, Inc., a Connecticut company, claims it has found a common pathway used by several viruses to infect host cells. The antiviral medications mimic the host cells and trick the virus to enter the drug rather than the host cell. The company is claiming that RabiCide™ was tested in animal trials in Vietnam with a high success rate against rabies. Detailed testing of this drug is not yet done in humans and no research articles have been published in scientific journals about it.

Researchers recently identified a novel protein that covers the rabies virus during its perilous journey in animal cells. The rabies viral RNA is protected by a nucleoprotein that makes it difficult for the human and animal immune systems to detect and destroy the virus. Specific drug systems may be able to target these proteins to make the rabies RNA vulnerable to attack by the host's immune system. This is an interesting idea yet to be tested in experiments.

Another target protein is the matrix protein of the lyssaviruses. The matrix protein links the viral envelope with its internal core. These proteins play a crucial role in the life cycle of the rabies virus. Its primary function is virus assembly and budding from the affected host cell. It is also involved in the regulation of the process of genetic building up of the new virions. The hope is that someday new treatments could be based on blocking the function of this critical protein.

RNA (Ribonucleic Acid) Interference

Brazilian researchers led by Brandao have recently published an exciting new way of counteracting rabies virus (Brandao et al., 2007). This is a very intricate concept of using short interfering RNAs (siRNAs). These are small segments of RNA that will interact with the replicating mechanisms of RNA to prevent its propagation. In experimental conditions, they were successful in reducing the level of rabies virus. It remains to be seen whether researchers can replicate these results in live animals. RNA interference can also have powerful applications because it can affect gene regulation. The concerns about this nascent technology include "off-target" effects on other similar-looking genes or proteins causing unpredictable side effects.

The Future of the Milwaukee Protocol

Scientists at the University of Wisconsin researched the topic and formulated a protocol that led to the first rabies survivor. Children's Hospital of Wisconsin in Milwaukee maintains a rabies directory for registering cases of rabies (Children's Hospital of Wisconsin, 2008). An exhaustive 58-page protocol can be downloaded from the site. This protocol painstakingly explains each of the steps to be taken to follow the protocol. Management of the patients with deliberately induced coma in the intensive care unit is extremely complicated, and the protocol spells out different options in case of various complications. An abbreviated five-page check list is also available at the website. This protocol is an evolving concept. The latest version (version 2.1) did not mandate the use of ribavirin. Originally ribavirin was used in the belief it would protect the heart against rabies. Ribavirin does not cross the blood-brain barrier if given only for a short period of time. Ribavirin can also cause complications such as the destruction of one's own blood (hemolysis). Because of these reasons, the scientists no longer strongly recommend ribavirin.

So far, seven patients were enrolled in the registry with no survivors. More data on mitochondrial toxicity associated with the treatment and the methods to treat it with a "mitochondrial cocktail" are available in the most recent protocol. The cases in which the protocol could be tried are going to be small, given the protocol's cost and complexity. Among the first ten attempts to replicate the Milwaukee Protocol, only two attempts met the two assumptions and included all of the four key drugs. None of the cases, including these two, survived. Attempts were done in Brazil (two), Canada, Germany (two), India, Thailand, and the United States (three). Overall, the total survival rate with the protocol is greater than the survival rate with the standard treatment for rabies. With usual treatments, patients survive for about 20 days. The Milwaukee Protocol, even when it failed to save the patients, increased the length of survival to about 70 days. This definitely gives hope for the future.

Questions for the Future

Rabies research raises several questions for the future. They are relevant on different levels. The foremost issue in sight is how can we control the vast number of deaths occurring in developing countries? Research in the developed world, such as the Milwaukee Protocol, which helped save a life, could not be replicated in developing countries because of its sophisticated nature and cost. It is ironic that these are the areas sorely in need of such interventions, with enough cases to test a new theory or modality of treatment. WHO and other international agencies have an important role to play in this regard.

There are also scientific questions in the rabies research field. As mentioned earlier, the exact pathophysiology of rabies in human beings is unknown. New leads have been discovered regarding the role of various neurotransmitters and receptors in rabies virus infection. Interestingly, different species (fox, dog, bat, etc.) are infected by specific types of lyssaviruses, the viruses responsible for rabies. The evolutionary history of these viruses is also not known. Why is the fox strain less pathogenic than the dog strain? Can the dynamics of the infection change over time? Will bat rabies become more common and emerge as a zoonosis in developed countries? Answers to these questions might provide freedom from rabies for humankind.

Abbreviations

AIDS	Acquired immune deficiency syndrome
BPL	Beta propiolactone
CDC	Centers for Disease Control and Prevention
CSF	Cerebrospinal fluid
DFA	Direct fluorescent antibody
dL	Deciliter
DNA	Deoxyribonucleic acid
EBLV	European bat *Lyssavirus*
EEG	Electroencephalogram
EU	European Union
FDA	Food and Drug Administration
HDCV	Human diploid cell vaccine
HIV	Human immunodeficiency virus
HRIG	Human rabies immune globulin
ICU	Intensive care unit
IgG	Immunoglobulin G
IU	International Units
km	Kilometer
ml	Milliliter

mm	Millimeter
MRI	Magnetic resonance imaging
NIH	National Institute of Health
ORV	Oral rabies vaccination
PCECV	Purified chick embryo cell vaccine
PCR	Polymerase chain reaction
PEP	Postexposure prophylaxis
RIG	Rabies immune globulin
RNA	Ribonucleic acid
RT-PCR	Reverse transcriptase polymerase chain reaction
RVA	Rabies vaccine adsorbed
SARS	Severe acute respiratory syndrome
UNICEF	United Nations Children's Fund
USDA	Untied States Department of Agriculture
WBC	White blood cell
WHO	World Health Organization

Glossary

Acetylcholine A chemical compound present in the nerve endings of various parts of the body enabling the nerve impulses to pass.

Acute Of sudden onset, as opposed to chronic, which means a condition that is present for a considerable period of time.

Adenovirus Medium-sized viruses without outer coverings, capable of producing several infections in humans including respiratory infections.

Adhesion molecules Molecules present on the surface of cells mediating the adhesion of other cells or microorganisms.

Aerophobia Fear of air, seen in rabies.

Aneurysm Abnormal enlargement of arteries (vessels carrying blood from the heart to the various parts of the body).

Angioneurotic edema Rapid swellings of the skin and mucosa that can result from a variety of causes, including side effects of drugs. The patient might develop breathing difficulties from swelling of the mucosa of the respiratory tract.

Antemortem Before death.

Antibiotics Chemical substances that kill microorganisms such as bacteria, fungi, or parasites.

Antibody A specific protein produced by the immune system in response to a specific foreign protein or particle called an antigen.

Anticoagulant A substance capable of preventing coagulation or clotting, thus causing uncontrolled bleeding.

Antigen A substance that can stimulate an immune reaction in the body. This reaction results in the production of antibody that will eventually combine with antigen and might neutralize the antigen by forming a complex.

Antiviral drugs Drugs effective against viruses.

Apoptosis Programmed cell death in which cells of a living organism decay or die themselves in response to various stimuli.

Arachnoid membrane The middle of the three coverings of the brain and spinal cord.

Artery Blood vessels carrying blood from the heart to different parts of the body.

Ataxia Unsteadiness in walking that indicates several neurological illnesses.

Bacteria Single-celled microorganisms that are ubiquitous.

Biologicals They are isolated from a variety of natural sources including human, animal, or microorganisms and include a wide range of products such as vaccines, blood, and blood components.

Biopsy A procedure by which a small sample of tissue is removed and studied for the purpose of diagnosis.

Bird flu Fatal influenza type seen in birds that can also affect humans, although rarely.

Blood pressure Force exerted on the blood vessel walls by the circulating blood. A low blood pressure indicates impairment of circulation and is a serious condition.

Brain swelling Swelling of the brain cells with water caused by a variety of stimuli including infections. This swelling results in impairment of function.

Brainstem Part of the brain connecting the forebrain and the spinal cord. Contains the centers controlling breathing and beating of the heart.

Canine distemper virus Highly contagious virus that attacks the respiratory, gastrointestinal, and nervous systems of dogs.

Cell culture Culture of layers of cells preserved in the laboratory; the cells are still living.

Cells Smallest structural and functional unit of all living organisms.

Cerebrospinal fluid (CSF) Clear body fluid seen below the middle layer of the coverings of the brain and spinal cord. Specific changes are noted in several diseases.

Cervical Pertaining to the neck.

Chemokine Protein secreted by cells instrumental in guiding other cells in migration.

Chronic Long standing.

Coma A profound state of unconsciousness caused by a variety of reasons.

Computed tomographic (CAT) scan X-ray technique used to show images of the inner parts of the body.

Cornea Transparent front portion of the eye with many nerve fibers and without any blood vessels.

Culture Method of growing microorganisms selectively in different mediums in the laboratory where they obtain nourishment.

Cytomegalovirus A virus belonging to the herpes virus family, causing infections predominantly in immunocompromised individuals.

Deciliter (dL) One-tenth of a liter.

Deoxyribonucleic acid (DNA) Chemical structure carrying the genetic information of an organism.

Diabetes mellitus Disease characterized by uncontrolled levels of glucose in the blood and urine.

Diagnosis The process of identifying a particular disease based on the external features, examination of the patient, and a review of the blood work.

Direct fluorescent antibody test Laboratory tests using a fluorescent dye to identify microorganisms.

Disorientation Altered behavior characterized by decreased orientation.

Dysphagia Difficulty in swallowing.

Empiric Practice based on experience, not necessarily on scientific experiments.

Encephalitis Swelling of the brain.

Encephalomyelitis Swelling of the brain and the spinal cord.

Endoplasmic reticulum Structure found inside a cell that has an important role in the production of proteins.

Endosome Compartments inside the cell important in the transportation of substances in the cell.

Enzootic Infection maintained in a particular animal species.

Enzyme Substances that catalyze chemical reactions.

Epidemic Spread of disease in large numbers.

Epidemiology Study about the factors affecting health and diseases.

Epitope A small portion of a larger protein or organism recognized by the body's immune system.

Epizootic A disease affecting many animals of one kind at the same time, especially in the wild.

F (Fahrenheit) A unit for measuring temperature.

Feral Stray animal without an owner.

Foramen magnum Opening at the lowest part of the skull through which the spinal cord continues downwards.

Gene A collection of different sequences capable of controlling the organism's development and structure.

Genome The information coded by DNA in an organism. It may contain gene and noncoding sequences.

Golgi bodies Stacks of membrane-covered sacs that package and move proteins to the outside of the cell.

Graft Tissue transferred from one site to another.

Guano Droppings of bats rich in nitrogen and phosphorous.

Guillain–Barré syndrome A disease in which the patient develops progressive weakness and numbness of all four limbs, possibly caused by an immune reaction to viral infections.

Hazmat suit A cloth that gives protection from hazardous materials.

Hepatitis Inflammation of the liver.

Hibernation State of prolonged inactivity (especially in winter) during which bats greatly reduce their normal metabolic activities.

Histopathological examination Methods of examining tissue samples under the microscope.

Human T-lymphotropic virus A type of virus capable of causing illnesses such as leukemia and weakness of legs.

Hybridoma Cells are fused with rapidly proliferating myeloma cells in the laboratory to augment the production of antibodies.

Hydrophobia Fear of water.

Hyperreflexia Increased reflexes indicating irritability of the nervous system.

Hypersalivation Increased amounts of salivation.

Hypertension Increased blood pressure.

Immune globulin Globulin made from pooled plasma of healthy volunteers capable of preventing several diseases.

Immunity Natural defenses of the body capable of preventing diseases.

Immunodeficiency Deficient immunity leading to susceptibility for several infections.

Immunoglobulin Antibody present in individuals with natural resistance to infections.

Immunology Branch of medical science dealing with body defenses.

Inoculation Introduction of vaccine or serum to an animal or human body.

Insomnia Lack of sleep.

Interferon Proteins produced by various cells in the body in response to several microorganisms.

Intracranially Inside the skull.

Intradermal Into the skin.

Intraperitoneally Inside the abdominal cavity.

Intron Noncoding regions of a gene.

Intubation Inserting a tube into the breathing pipe to facilitate breathing.

Lagomorphs An order of mammals that includes hares and rabbits.

Liver Large organ in the abdomen which has several functions including clearing toxins from the body.

Lumbar puncture (spinal tap) A procedure in which a long, thin needle is inserted between the vertebrae in a person's spine to remove a sample of cerebrospinal fluid.

Lyme disease An emerging infectious disease spread through tick bites.

Lymphocyte A type of blood cells important in body defenses.

Lyssavirus A genus of viruses belonging to the family of *Rhabdoviridae*.

Macrophage Large cells important in defense from infections.

Magnetic resonance imaging Newer type of imaging modality used to define structure and functions of various body parts.

Malaria Infection common in tropics transmitted by mosquitoes.

Meningitis Serious infection of the coverings of the brain.

Meningoencephalitis Combination of inflammation of the covering of the brain (meningitis) and the brain.

Microliter (μL) One one-thousandth of a milliliter (10^{-6} L). This is the same as a cubic millimeter.

Microscope An instrument used to enlarge and visualize small structures such as microorganisms.

Monoclonal antibodies Single type of antibody produced by cells of the same type.

Morbidity The burden, incidence, or prevalence of a disease.

Myeloma A type of serious cancer caused by the unlimited proliferation of plasma cells that help in body defenses.

Necropsy Examination of a dead animal.

Negri bodies Pink inclusion body seen in rabies virus-affected brains.

Nephrotic syndrome Disease of kidneys characterized by excessive loss of protein through the urine.

Neuron The basic cell in the nervous system.

Neutrophils Type of blood cells important in body defenses.

Nuchal Pertaining to the neck.

Nucleocapsid The combination of the viral genome and its covering.

Obtundation Reduced level of alertness.

Oculocephalic reflexes A movement of eyes that could be shown even if the patient is unconscious. Absence might indicate severe damage of the brain.

Olfactory Cranial nerve running from the nose to the brain, helping in the sense of smell.

Paresthesia Abnormal sensation.

Pathogenicity Ability of an organism to cause a disease.

Peptide Compounds containing two or more amino acids. In turn, peptides can form proteins.

Peripheral nerves The nerve fibers originating from the spinal cord and supplying various body parts.

Phagocytic activity The act of ingesting microorganisms or proteins.

Pharyngitis Inflammation of the pharynx.

Pia mater The covering of the brain that is closest to the brain.

Placebo Sham or dummy pills used in clinical research work.

Plasma Yellow-colored liquid portions of the blood.

Plasmid Small circular DNAs that can replicate in the bacteria.

Pneumococcus Microorganisms that can cause severe pneumonia in an adult.

Pneumonia Infection of the lung, usually caused by bacteria.

Polymerase An enzyme that is vital in the replication process of DNA.

Polymerase chain reaction Technique used in the laboratory to amplify the presence of small amounts of genetic material.

Polysaccharide Long chains of sugar molecules combined together.

Postexposure prophylaxis Prevention of the disease after one is exposed to the disease.

Pre-exposure prophylaxis Prevention of the disease before one is exposed.

Prevalence Number of cases of the disease in the population.

Prodromal phase Early part of the disease when the patient still has vague or nonspecific symptoms.

Prodrome Early nonspecific symptoms at the beginning of a disease.

Prognosis Knowledge or prediction of the fate of a disease.

Prolapsed vertebral disk Slippage of the vertebral disk (structure interposed between the vertebrae or the back bones) from its normal place.

Prophylaxis Prevention of a disease using a drug or a vaccine.

Pupils Small opening in the eye that reacts to the amount of light shone into the eye.

Quarantine A period in which a person or animal suspected of carrying a disease is detained at the port of entry to a country to prevent the spread of the disease.

Radiculopathy Involvement of the nerves coming out of the spinal cord causing symptoms such as numbness and weakness.

Receptors A protein usually present on the cell surface that binds to a specific molecule.

Recombinant technology Technique by which a gene from one animal is combined with gene from another to produce large quantities of purified substances such as proteins.

Reflex An involuntary response to a stimuli mediated by the nerves in the body.

Respirator (ventilator) Machine that helps a patient to breathe.

Respiratory failure Inability to provide enough oxygen to the body so that the person might stop breathing completely soon.

Reverse transcriptase polymerase chain reaction (RT-PCR) Two-step procedure by which RNA can be converted into DNA in the laboratory.

Ribonucleic acid This is made of a chain of nucleotides, similar to DNA, but has only one chain instead of the two as in DNA.

Seizure Convulsions

Sensorium Level of consciousness and the way an individual is reacting to the surroundings.

Simian Related to monkeys.

siRNA Short interfering RNA.

Spinal cord Long tubular bundle of nerves starting from the brain, extending along the back, and supplying nerves to all four limbs.

Steroids Chemicals found in plants and animals with a variety of actions and also used widely as drugs for different conditions.

Strychnine A poison used to kill vampire bats.

Subarachnoid hemorrhage Bleeding into the space under the arachnoid membrane that covers the spinal cord and brain.

Supraorbital Above the eyes.

Sylvatic Disease cycle that affects only wild animals.

Syphilis A sexually transmitted disease that can affect various organs of the body including the nervous system.

Taeniafuge An agent or medicine for expelling tapeworms from the body.

Tissue A group of cells that perform the same function in unison.

Toxoplasmosis Disease caused by a parasite that is more common in patients with organ transplants.

Transgenic plants Plants carrying a gene transferred from other living beings.

Transplant An organ being moved from one body to another.

Transplantation Procedure of moving an organ or tissue from one body to another.

Vaccine A preparation used to improve immunity to a specific disease.

Vaccinia virus Originally used for immunization against smallpox.

Vector An animal or insect that carries a disease-producing organism.

Virion An individual particle of the virus.

Virus Tiny infectious agents unable to grow outside a living cell and requiring cells for their survival and propagation.

Vocal cord Bands or folds of mucous membrane in the throat helping in speech.

West Nile virus A viral disease that can cause several manifestations including swelling of the brain. Introduced in the western hemisphere in 1999.

White blood cell (WBC) The blood cell important in the defense against infecting microorganisms, also known as leukocytes.

Zoonosis Any disease of animals that can be transmitted to humans. Rabies is an example of a zoonosis.

Bibliography

Alvarez L. et al. 1994. Partial Recovery from Rabies in a Nine-Year-Old Boy. *Pediatr Infect Dis J* 13:1154–5.

American Society for Microbiology. 1997. The Scientific Future of DNA for Immunization.

Anonymous. Egypt to Resume Shooting of Stray Dogs. *The Australian*, October 1, 2007. Accessed on May 11, 2008, at http://www.theaustralian.news.com.au/story/0,25197,22510493-12377,00.html.

Anonymous. Jefferson Scientists Create Tobacco Plant to Produce Antibodies Against Rabies. *Science Daily*, June 4, 2003.

Anonymous. The Newark Dog Scare; Plenty of Money to Send the Children to Paris. *New York Times*, December 6, 1885.

Bat Conservation International. 2008. *Natural History of Bats*. Accessed on May 12, 2008, at http://www.batcon.org/home/index.asp?idPage=121.

BBC News. 2002. *Rabies Confirmed in Bat Worker* [Online November 2002]. Accessed on May 12, 2008, at http://news.bbc.co.uk/1/hi/scotland/2508043.stm.

Brandao, P.E. et al. 2007. Short-Interfering RNAs as Antivirals Against Rabies. *Braz J Infect Dis* 11:224–5.

CDC. 1983a. Epidemiologic Notes and Reports Human Rabies—Michigan. *Morb Mortal Wkly Rep* 32(12):159–60.

CDC. 1983b. Human Rabies – Kenya. *Morb Mortal Wkly Rep*. 32:494-5. Accessed on May 12, 2008, at http://www.cdc.gov/mmwr/preview/mmwrhtml/00000146.htm.

CDC. 1986. Epidemiologic Notes and Reports Rabies in a Javelina—Arizona. *Morb Mortal Wkly Rep* 35(35):555–6.

CDC. 1995. Mass Treatment of Humans Exposed to Rabies—New Hampshire, 1994. *Morb Mortal Wkly Rep* 44:484–6.

CDC. 1996. Human Rabies—Connecticut, 1995. *Morb Mortal Wkly Rep* 45(10):207–9.

CDC. 1998. Notice to Readers Availability of New Rabies Vaccine for Human Use. *Morb Mortal Wkly Rep.* 47:12. Accessed on May 4, 2008, at http://www.cdc.gov/mmwr/preview/mmwrhtml/00050848.htm.

CDC. 1999. Human Rabies Prevention—United States, 1999. Recommendations of the Advisory Committee on Immunization Practices (ACIP). *Morb Mortal Wkly Rep* 48(RR-1):1–21.

CDC. 2000. BMBL Section III. *Laboratory Biosafety Level Criteria* [Online 2000]. Accessed on May 12, 2008, at http://www.cdc.gov/od/ohs/biosfty/bmbl4/bmbl4s3.htm.

CDC. 2003. Human Death Associated with Bat Rabies–California. *Morb Mortal Wkly Rep* 53(2):33–5.

CDC. 2004. Investigation of Rabies Infections in Organ Donor and Transplant Recipients—Alabama, Arkansas, Oklahoma, and Texas, 2004. *Morb Mortal Wkly Rep* 53:586–9.

CDC. 2005a. Compendium of Animal Rabies Prevention and Control. *Morb Mortal Wkly Rep* 54:1–8. Accessed on May 12, 2008, at http://www.cdc.gov/mmwr/preview/mmwrhtml/rr5403a1.htm.

CDC. 2005b. Human Rabies—Mississippi. *Morb Mortal Wkly Rep.* 55(8):207–8.

CDC. 2006. Human Rabies—Indiana and California. *Morb Mortal Wkly Rep* 56: 361–365.

CDC. 2007a. *What Does Rabies Preexposure Prophylaxis Involve?* [Online September 2007]. Accessed on May 5, 2008, at http://www.cdc.gov/rabies/exposure/preexposure.html.

CDC. 2007b. *What to Do if You Have a Potential Rabies Exposure* [Online September 2007]. Accessed on May 5, 2008, at http://www.cdc.gov/rabies/exposure/types.html.

CDC. 2007c. *What Does Rabies Preexposure Prophylaxis Involve?* Accessed on April 17, 2008, at http://www.cdc.gov/rabies/exposure/preexposure.html.

CDC. 2007d. *Bats and Rabies* [Online July 2007]. Accessed on May 5, 2008, at http://www.cdc.gov/rabies/bats.html.

CDC. 2008a. *Prevention of Specific Infectious Diseases* [Online May 2008]. Accessed on May 12, 2008, at http://wwwn.cdc.gov/travel/yellowBookCh4-Rabies.aspx.

CDC. 2008b. *About Rabies* [Online July 2007]. Accessed on May 12, 2008, at http://www.cdc.gov/rabies/about.html.

CDC. 2008c. *Protocol for Postmortem Diagnosis of Rabies in Animals by Direct Fluorescent Antibody Testing.* Accessed on May 12, 2008, at http://www.cdc.gov/rabies/docs/standard_dfa_protocol_rabies.pdf.

CDC. 2008d. Public Health Response to a Rabid Kitten—Four States, 2007. *Morb Mortal Wkly Rep* 56:1337–40.

Chang, Hwa-Gan. 2002. Public Health Impact of Reemergence of Rabies, New York. *Emerg Infect Dis* 8:909–13.

Children's Hospital of Wisconsin. 2008. *Rabies Registry Home Page* [Online 2008] Accessed on May 12, 2008, at http://www.chw.org/display/PPF/DocID/33223/router.asp.

CIWEC Clinic Travel Medicine Center. 2007. *Risk of rabies in Nepal* [Online August 2007]. Accessed on July 27, 2008, at http://www.ciwec-clinic.com/immune/rabies.html.

Clark, Keith A. *Rabies from Cats*. From the Zoonosis Control Division, Texas Department of Health, May 15, 1988. Accessed on April 22, 2008, at http://www.avma.org/reference/zoonosis/znrabies.asp.

Crucell. 2006. *Rabies Antibody Cocktail* [Online 2006]. Accessed on May 12, 2008, at http://www.crucell.com/R_and_D-Clinical_Development-Rabies_Antibody_Product.

da Rosa et al. 2006. Bat-transmitted Human Rabies Outbreaks, Brazilian Amazon. *Emerging Infectious Diseases*. 12:1197.

Department for Environment, Food, and Rural Affairs. 2008. *Bringing Pets to the UK* [Online, May 2008]. Accessed on May 12, 2008, at http://www.defra.gov.uk/animalh/quarantine/index.htm.

Dolan, Jr., Edward F. 1958. *Pasteur and the Invisible Giants*. New York: Dodd, Mead and Company.

European Commission. 2002. *The Oral Vaccination of Foxes against Rabies*. Accessed on April 18 2008, at http://ec.europa.eu/food/fs/sc/scah/out80_en.pdf.

Fox News. 2006. *Nearly 1,000 Virginia Girl Scouts Urged to Get Rabies Shots*. Accessed on April 20, 2008, at http://www.foxnews.com/story/0,2933,207204,00.html.

Geison, Gerald L. 1995. *The Private Science of Louis Pasteur*. Princeton: Princeton University Press.

Georgia Department of Human Resources. 2004. *Cures for Human Rabies: Superstition to Science*. Accessed on May 12, 2008, at http://health.state.ga.us/healthtopics/mme/042604.asp.

Gilmore, Robert. 1995. The Healing Tradition. *OzarksWatch* vol. 3, no. 1. Accessed on May 12, 2008, at http://thelibrary.org/lochist/periodicals/ozarkswatch/ow801c.htm.

Gipson, Fred. 1990. *Old Yeller*. New York: HarperCollins.

Greenhall, Arthur M. 1968. Problems and Ecological Implications in the Control of Vampire Bats. Proc. IUCN Latin Amer. Conf. Conservation Renewable Natural Resources. *San Carlos Bariloche*, Argentina, 27 March–2 April 1968, pp. 94–102. Accessed on May 5, 2008, at http://digitalcommons.unl.edu/cgi/viewcontent.cgi?article=1012&context=vpcfour.

Hattwick. M.A.W. et al. 1972. Recovery from Rabies: A Case Report. *Ann Intern Med* 76:931–42.

Health Protection Agency. 2005. Case of Imported Rabies in the UK. *Communicable Disease Report Weekly* 15(30): News.

Health Protection Agency. 2006. Rabies in Patients Who Received Organ Transplants in Germany. *Communicable Disease Report Weekly* 16(51):News.

Henahan, Sean. 1997. *DNA Vaccine Outlook*. Access Excellence [Online 2007]. Accessed on May 12, 2008, at http://www.accessexcellence.org/WN/SUA11/dnavax1297.php.

Hendekli, C.M. 2005. Current Therapies in Rabies. *Arch Virol* 150: 1047–57.

Hu, W.T. et al. 2007. Long-Term Follow-up after Treatment of Rabies by Induction of Coma. *N Engl J Med* 357:945–6.

Jackson, Alan C. 1994. The Fatal Neurologic Illness of the Fourth Duke of Richmond in Canada: Rabies. *Ann R Coll Phys Surg Can* 27:40–41.

Jackson, Alan C. 2000. Rabies. *Can J Neurol Sci* 27:278–83.

Jackson, Alan C. 2005. Recovery from Rabies. *N Engl J Med* 352:2549–2550.

Jackson, Alan C., and William H. Wunner, eds. 2002. *Rabies*. San Diego: Academic Press.

Jackson, Alan C. et al. 2003. Management of Rabies in Humans. *Clin Infect Dis* 36:60–3.

Judson, Olivia. A Coffin for Rabies. *The New York Times*. January 15, 2008. Accessed May 12, 2008, at http://judson.blogs.nytimes.com/2008/01/15/a-coffin-for-rabies/index.html?ex=1358744400&en=16b4b960b24d59bb&ei=5088&partner=rssnyt&emc= rss.

Krause, R. et al. 2005. Travel-associated Rabies in Austrian Man. *Emerg Infect Dis* 11:719.

Ladogana, A. et al. 1994. Modification of Tritiated Gamma-Amino-n-Butyric Acid Transport in Rabies Virus-Infected Primary Cortical Cultures. *J Gen Virol* 75:623–7.

Licata, J.M. and Harty, R.N. 2003. Rhabdoviruses and Apoptosis. *Int Rev Immunol* 22:451–76.

Mackowiak, Philip A. 2007. *Post Mortem: Solving History's Great Medical Masteries*. Philadelphia: American College of Physicians.

Madhusudana, S.N. et al. 2002. Partial Recovery from Rabies in a Six-Year-Old Girl. *Int J Infect Dis* 6:85–6.

Massachusetts Department of Public Health. 2004. *Rabies Scenarios: Living with Rabies in Your Community* [Online July 2004]. Accessed on May 12, 2008, at http://www.mass.gov/Eeohhs2/docs/dph/cdc/rabies/rabies_scenarios.pdf.

Matsumoto, S. 1963. Electron Microscope Studies of Rabies Virus in Mouse Brain. *J Cell Biol* 19:565–91.

Molecular Targeting Technologies. 2008. *Rabies Monoclonal Antibody Product* [Online 2008]. Accessed on May 12, 2008, at http://www.mtarget.com/pdfs/pipeline/Rabies MonoclonalAnti.pdf.

New York Times. The Newark Dog Scare, December 6, 1885.

North Carolina Public Health. 2008. *Preventing Spread of Raccoon Rabies, West of North Carolina: Oral Rabies Vaccine Program* [Online 2008]. Accessed on May 11, 2008, at http://www.epi.state.nc.us/epi/rabies/orv1.html.

Parker, James N. and Parker, Philip M. 2002. *The Official Patient's Sourcebook on Rabies*. San Diego: ICON Group International.

Porras, C. et al. 1976. Recovery from Rabies in a Man. *Ann Intern Med* 85:44–8.

Real, E. et al. 2004. Antiviral Drug Discovery Strategy Using Combinatorial Libraries of Structurally Constrained Peptides. *J Virol* 78:7410–7.

Robbins, A. et al. 2005. Bat Incidents at Children's Camps, New York State, 1998–2002. *Emerg Infect Dis* 11:302–5.

Robbins, Louise E. 2001. *Louis Pasteur and the Hidden World of Microbes*. Oxford: Oxford University Press.

Rupprecht, C.E. and Gibbons, R.V. 2004. Clinical Practice. Prophylaxis Against Rabies. *N Engl J Med* 351:2626–35.

Rupprecht, C.E. et al. 1995. The Ascension of Wildlife Rabies: A Cause for Public Health Concern or Intervention? *Emerg Infect Dis* 1:107–14.

Sandeep, K. Man's Worst Foe. *The Hindu*, May 6, 2002.

Schmiedel, S. et al. 2007. Case report on fatal human rabies infection in Hamburg, Germany, March 2007. *Euro Surveill* 12(5):E070531.5.

Schweighardt, B. and Atwood, W.J. 2001. Virus Receptors in the Human Central Nervous System. *J Neurovirol* 7:187–95.

Solomon, T. et al. 2005. Paralytic Rabies after a Two Week Holiday in India. *BMJ* 331:501–503.

Srinivasan, A. et al. 2005. Transmission of Rabies Virus from an Organ Donor to Four Transplant Recipients. *N Engl J Med* 352 (11): 1103–11.

Stanley, George F.G. 2000. *Dictionary of Canadian Biography Online.* Lennox, Charles, 4th Duke of Richmond and Lennox. Accessed on April 17, 2008, at http://www.biographi. ca/EN/ShowBio.asp?BioId=36622.

Texas Department of State Health Services 2004, *Rabies in Texas: A Historical Perspective.* Accessed on April 20, 2008, at http://www.dshs.state.tx.us/idcu/disease/rabies/ history/historyInTexas.pdf.

Tillotson, J.R. et al. 1977. Rabies in a Laboratory Worker–New York. *Morb Mortal Wkly Rep* 26:183–4.

van Thiel, P.P. et al. 2008. Fatal Case of Human Rabies (Duvenhage Virus) from a Bat in Kenya: The Netherlands, December 2007. *Euro Surveill.* 13: 8007.

Virginia Department of Health. 2006. *2006 Press Releases.* Accessed on May 12, 2008, at http://www.vdh.state.va.us/news/PressReleases/2007/index.htm.

Wandeler, A.I. et al. 1988. Oral Immunization of Wildlife Against Rabies: Concept and First Field Experiments. *Rev Infect Dis* 10 Suppl 4:S649–53.

Warrell, D.A. 1976. The Clinical Picture of Rabies in Man. *Trans R Soc Trop Med Hyg* 70:188–95.

Warrell, M.J., and Warrell, D.A. 2004. Rabies and other Lyssavirus diseases. *Lancet* 363:959–69.

WHO. 2002. *Current WHO Guide for Rabies Pre and Post-Exposure Treatment in Human* [Online November 2002]. Accessed on May 5, 2008, at http://www.who.int/rabies/ en/WHO_guide_rabies_pre_post_exp_treat_humans.pdf.

WHO. 2005. *WHO Technical Report Series 931. WHO Expert Consultation on Rabies, First Report* [Online 2005]. Accessed on May 11, 2008, at http://www.who.int/ rabies/trs931_%2006_05.pdf.

WHO. 2008a. *Rabies* [Online 2008] Accessed on May 12, 2008, at http://www.who.int/ topics/rabies/en/.

WHO. 2008b. Welcome to Rabnet [Online 2008]. Accessed on May 12, 2008, at http://www.who.int/globalatlas/default.asp.

WHO. 2008c. *Virus Identification Using Monoclonal Antibodies* [Online 2008]. Accessed on May 12, 2008, at https://www.who.int/rabies/human/virus_identification/en/.

Williams, Lisa M. and Brittingham, Margaret. 2006. *A Homeowner's Guide to Northeastern Bats and Bat Problems.* University Park: The Pennsylvania State University. Accessed on July 28, 2008, at https://pubs.cas.psu.edu/FreePubs/pdfs/uh081.pdf.

Willoughby, R.E. et al. 2005. Survival after Treatment of Rabies with Induction of Coma. *N Engl J Med* 352:2508–2514.

World Rabies Day. 2008. *World Rabies Day Mission* [Online 2008]. Accessed on May 12, 2008, at http://www.worldrabiesday.org/EN/World_Rabies_Day_Mission.html.

Xiang, Zhiquan et al. 2002. Novel, Chimpanzee Serotype 68-Based Adenoviral Vaccine Carrier for Induction of Antibodies to a Transgene Product. *J Virol* 76:2667–75.

Index

About the Author

P. DILEEP KUMAR is an internal medicine physician with several years of experience. He has published more than 90 papers in various peer reviewed scientific journals and presented papers in several medical conferences. Dr. Kumar is a peer reviewer for several international medical journals. He is also active in the American College of Physicians, serving in various capacities, including judging presentations at the regional and national meetings.